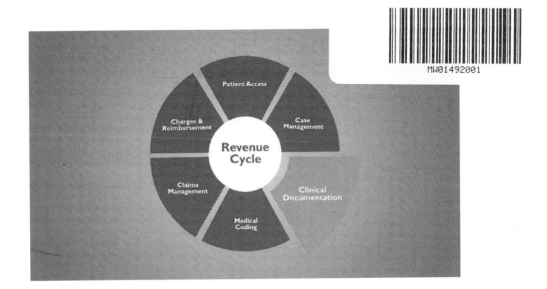

MRA/HCC CHART REVIEW & DOCUMENTATION GUIDE

A Brief Step-By-Step Guide on Chart Audits for Optimal Risk Adjustment Captures

HCCs (Hierarchical Condition Categories) were designed as a risk adjustment system to facilitate reimbursement models based on predicted healthcare service expenditures. This guide will help provide tips on where many relevant HCC ICD-10 Codes can be found within a chart/records to assist Coders & Providers to look for such conditions relevant to Medicare Risk Adjustment capture.

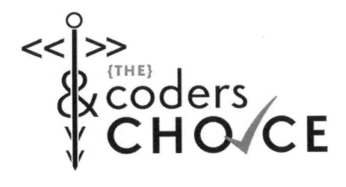

<<|>>
{THE}
&coders
CHOICE

TABLE OF CONTENTS

CMS MEDICAL RECORD GUIDANCE

Criteria for CMS Validation Audits

- ➤ MUST include the patient name, date of birth, and date of encounter
- ➤ MUST be a face-to-face visit
- ➤ Must be a valid provider (Physician, Nurse Practitioner, Physician Assistant)
- ➤ MUST be a legible note with no abbreviations or symbols, such as up or down arrows
- ➤ MUST be signed by the provider with full name and credentials in legible form
- ➤ MUST have an authenticated signature validation (Handwritten or Electronic)
- ➤ MUST address all of the diagnoses used in the clinical decision making for the visit
- ➤ MUST clearly and specifically document the diagnoses in the encounter note with M.E.A.T. (Monitor, Evaluate, Assess, Treat) criteria
- ➤ MUST contain ALL elements of a S.O.A.P. (Subjective, Objective, Assessment, Plan) note
  - ○ Subjective
    - ▪ Chief Complaint
    - ▪ History of Present Illness (HPI)
  - ○ Objective
    - ▪ Vitals Signs
    - ▪ Labs
    - ▪ Physical Exam
  - ○ Assessment
    - ▪ Sometimes referred to as "Impression"
    - ▪ Lists the diagnoses (ICD-10 Codes)
  - ○ Plan
    - ▪ Should state clearly what the treatment will be for each condition listed under the Assessment/Impression
      - • Example: COPD (J44.9) – The patient is currently being treated with Spiriva and will be followed by Pulmonology)
  - ○ All progress notes should be signed and closed within 72 hours and always prior to claims submission as a condition of payment.

DOCUMENTATION GUIDELINES SUMMARY

- ➢ Include on every page:
    1) Patient's complete name
    2) Unique Identifier
        - Date of Birth and/or Medical Record Number
        - Date of Service
        - Page Number
- ➢ Documentation Characteristics:
    1) Clear
    2) Concise
    3) Consistent
    4) Complete
    5) Legible
- ➢ Follow S.O.A.P. Format:
    1) S: Subjective
        - Chief Complaint
            - How the Patient described the problem
        - History of Present Illness
            - Combines the recent history, as delivered by the patient, of their illness with input from the physician
            - Has replaced the traditional "Subjective" portion
            - Very important because it is where you can and should document much of the evaluation and assessment of each diagnosis listed later in the "Assessment" or "Impression" portion of the note
    2) O: Objective
        - Data obtained from examination, lab results, vital signs, etc.
    3) A: Assessment
        - List of patient's current conditions and status of all chronic conditions
            - Examples:
                - CHF – Compensated

       o   COPD – Noted on CXR

       o   Major Depression – Improving on Meds

       o   Diabetes Mellitus – Diet Controlled

       o   Diabetic Neuropathy – Taking Gabapentin

4) P: Plan of Care

- Next steps in diagnosing problem further, prescriptions, consultations, referrals, patient education and recommended time to return for follow-up

➢ Signature Requirements:

1) All written progress notes should be signed by the provider. The signature should be handwritten. Stamps are NOT acceptable.

2) All dictated progress notes must be signed by the provider. The signature may be handwritten or electronic. Stamps are NOT acceptable.

3) All electronic medical record (EMR) progress notes should be closed and signed with a digital or an acceptable electronic signature:

- Acceptable EMR signature Examples:
  - "Electronically signed by…"
  - "Authenticated by…"
  - Validated by…"

4) Nurse practitioners and physician assistants may render service and MUST sign the progress notes

➢ Provider Credentials:

1) In addition to a signature, the provider's full name and credentials should be typed, printed or stamped on each progress note.

CHART AUDIT/REVIEW PROTOCOL

(Finding Potential HCC Codes)

> ## BMI:
> - o Look at BMI in the physical exam
>   - ▪ If the BMI is 40 or above, code Z68.4- and if provider documents "morbid obesity", can also code E66.01
>   - ▪ If the BMI is 35 or above and the patient has a comorbid condition, the provider can be queried to code E66.01 (Morbid Obesity)
>   - ▪ If the BMI is 30 or above and the patient has a diagnosis of obstructive sleep apnea (uses a CPAP), then E66.2 (Morbid Obesity with Alveolar Hypoventilation) can be queried for the provider to consider

> ## Depression Screening:
> - o During most MRA visits, there is a PHQ-9 Depression Screening done
> - o If there is a positive score for Major Depression (score of 15 or greater), then code the appropriate F-Code for Major Depressive Disorder (MDD)
>   - ▪ Interpretation of Total Score for Depression Severity (PHQ-9)
>   - • 1-4 Minimal depression
>   - • 5-9 Mild depression
>   - • 10-14 Moderate depression
>   - • 15-19 Moderately severe depression
>   - • 20-27 Severe depression

> ## Medications:
> - o Look for any insulin (Levemir, Humalog, Humulin, Novolog, Novolin)
>   - ▪ Code Z79.4 (HCC Category 19 – Diabetes without Complication)
> - o Look for any Diabetes medication (i.e. Metformin, Glucophage)

- Finding a diabetic medication in the medication list will trigger the coder to keep an eye out for a possible diabetes diagnosis for the patient, or at least query the provider if the diagnosis exists for the patient
  - Look for any opioid or benzodiazepine medications that are taken in high doses and for long periods of time (HCC 55 or 56 – Substance Use Disorders)
    - Opioids: OxyContin, Percocet, oxycodone, hydrocodone dependence (F11.20)
    - Xanax, alprazolam, Diazepam, Valium, clonazepam (F13.20)
  - Look for any familiar Depression medications (HCC 59, Major Depressive, Bipolar & Paranoid Disorders)
    - Abilify, Lexapro, Celexa, Escitalopram, Zoloft, Wellbutrin, Sertraline, Lithium
  - Look for any medication(s) that are chemotherapeutic agents used for cancer treatment, as it can be supporting evidence for a provider coding an active cancer
    - Doxorubicin (Adriamycin)
  - Gabapentin
    - If medication is given, can query provider for G63 (Polyneuropathy in diseases classified elsewhere) – HCC 75
    - If patient is diabetic, can indicate potential Diabetes with Neuropathy or Polyneuropathy (E11.40 or E11.42) – HCC 18

> **Past Medical History:**
  - Any past medical history listed conditions need supporting documentation to verify that the condition is still active
  - However, certain conditions do not need supporting documentation and are considered "status" conditions
    - Lower extremity toe or foot amputation (HCC 189 – Amputation Status)
    - Dialysis status (HCC 134 – Dialysis Status), which is ICD-10 Code Z99.2
  - Patients with a Past History of Drug or Alcohol Abuse/Dependence can be coded as "in remission"
    - Alcohol Dependence, in remission (F10.21) – HCC 55
    - Opioid Dependence, in remission (F11.21) – HCC 55

- o Patients with a Past History of Major Depression/Depressive Disorder can be coded as "in remission"
    - Major Depressive Disorder, recurrent, in remission (F33.40) – HCC 58
    - Major Depressive Disorder, recurrent, in partial remission (F33.41) – HCC 58

- ➢ **Social History:**
  - o Many Electronic Medical Record programs contain a "Drugs/Alcohol" screening in the social history portion of an MRA visit and inquire as to whether the patient uses or takes alcohol, drugs (Marijuana)
    - Alcohol Dependence, uncomplicated (F10.20) – HCC 55
    - Cannabis Dependence, uncomplicated (F12.20) – HCC 55
    - Cocaine Dependence, uncomplicated (F14.20) – HCC 55
  - o The social history may also provide information if there is a past history of any illicit drug use or alcohol abuse, which would then allow for query into a "remission" ICD-10 code to be used
    - Alcohol Dependence, in remission (F10.21) – HCC 55
    - Cannabis Dependence, in remission (F12.21) – HCC 55
    - Cocaine Dependence, in remission (F14.21) – HCC 55

- ➢ **Physical Examination:**
  - o Lower Extremities
    - Possible amputations (HCC 189)
    - Possible ulcers (HCC 157 or 158)
  - o Abdomen/Pelvis
    - Possible –ostomy (HCC 188 – Artificial Openings for Feeding or Elimination)
  - o Upper Extremities
    - Possible AV Fistula (HCC 108 – Vascular Disease)
    - They are commonly done in the arm, but on certain occasions it can be done in the legs, so it could also potentially be found in the lower extremities
  - o Late-Effects of CVA

- If a patient had a recent stroke or cerebrovascular accident, there is a potential for a late-effect condition, such as facial, left or right-sided weakness, etc.
  - Monoplegia of upper limb following cerebral infarction (I69.33-)
  - Monoplegia of lower limb following cerebral infarction (I69.34-)
  - Hemiplegia and hemiparesis following cerebral infarction (I69.35-)
  - Other paralytic syndrome following cerebral infarction (I69.36-)

- ➢ **Labs:**
  - Check the CBC (Complete Blood Count)
    - Platelet Count
      - If low, Thrombocytopenia (D69.6) – HCC 48
      - If high, Thrombocytosis (D47.3) – HCC 48
    - Absolute Neutrophil Count
      - If low, Neutropenia (D70.9) – HCC 47
  - Check the CMP (Comprehensive Metabolic Panel)
    - eGFR (estimated Glomerular Filtration Rate)
      - 30-59 (Chronic Kidney Disease, Stage 3) – HCC 138
      - 15-29 (Chronic Kidney Disease, Stage 4) – HCC 137
      - <15 (Chronic Kidney Disease, Stage 5 or End-Stage Renal Disease) – HCC 136
        - Patient may also be on dialysis (Z99.2)
    - Glucose
      - If patient is diabetic, elevated glucose levels for at least the last few labs done can indicate Type 2 Diabetes with Hyperglycemia (E11.65) – HCC 18 – Diabetes with Complications
  - HbA1c
    - Test done to detect diabetes
      - Below 5.7 % (Normal)
      - 5.7% to 6.4% (Prediabetes)

- 6.5% or greater (Diabetes)
  - o Parathyroid Hormone (PTH)
    - The Parathyroid Gland controls the calcium levels in the blood
    - If calcium levels are too high or too low, a PTH test can be done to see if the hormone levels are abnormal
    - Patients with Chronic Kidney Disease (CKD) can have derangements of their calcium levels, which can cause hyperparathyroidism, and a PTH will show abnormality, suggestive of Hyperparathyroidism of Renal Origin (N25.81) – HCC 23 – Other Significant Endocrine or Metabolic Disorders
    - Providers can be queried as to whether a PTH was or will be done if the patient has CKD

- ➢ **Radiological Exams:**
  - o Chest X-Ray
    - Incidental finding of Atherosclerosis of the Aorta, or Calcification of the Aorta (I70.0)
      - HCC 108
    - Thoracic Aortic Aneurysm (I71.2)
      - HCC 108
    - Thoracic Aortic Ectasia (I77.810)
      - HCC 108
    - Chronic Obstructive Pulmonary Disease (J44.9)
      - HCC 111
    - Pulmonary Fibrosis (J84.10) or Interstitial Pulmonary/Lung Disease (J84.9)
      - HCC 112
  - o Cervical, Thoracic, or Lumbar/Lumbosacral (X-Ray, CT or MRI)
    - Inflammatory Spondylopathy/Facet Arthropathy (M46.92, M46.84, M46.96, M46.97)
      - HCC 40
    - Impingement or Nerve Root Compression (G95.20, G95.29, G95.89)

- ICD-10 Codes are unspecified and other, so provider would have to document more specific details regarding the condition for capture requirements
- HCC 72

- Abdominal/Pelvic (X-Ray, Ultrasound, CT, MRI)
  - Abdominal Aortic Aneurysm (I71.4)
    - HCC 108
  - Atherosclerosis or Stenosis of Renal Artery (I70.1)
    - HCC 108
  - Disorder of Adrenal Gland (E27.9)
    - HCC 23
    - If a nodule or mass is seen
- Lower Extremity Ultrasound (Arterial)
  - Atherosclerosis of Native Arteries of the Extremities
    - I70.201 (Right Leg)
    - I70.202 (Left Leg)
    - I70.203 (Bilateral Legs)
    - I70.208 (Other Extremity)
    - I70.209 (Unspecified Extremity)
- Echocardiogram
  - Pulmonary Hypertension (I27.20)
    - HCC 85
- Brain (CT or MRI)
  - Benign Neoplasm of Brain, Meninges, or Spinal Cord (D32-D33)
    - HCC 12
    - Benign Neoplasms (D-Codes), are not HCC Codes, except for the brain and spinal cord locations

CODING SCENARIOS

Coding Scenario 1

Patient Name: Jane Doe	**Electronically Signed:** Dr. John Doe, D.O.
DOB: 05/21/1953	**Appt. Date/Time:** 4/5/2019
Insurance: Medicare Advantage (HMO)	**Appt. Type:** MCE

Chief Complaint: Follow up hyperlipidemia, HTN, OA, MDD

Vitals

BP: 134/71 sitting L arm	**BP Cuff Size:** adult	**Pulse:** 61 bpm regular
T: 97.8F oral	**O2Sat:** 93% RA	**Ht:** 62 in
W: 200lbs	**BMI:** 36.6	

ROS

Patient reports no frequent nosebleeds, no nose problems, and no sinus problems: congestion. She reports dry mouth but reports no sore throat, no bleeding gums, no snoring, no mouth ulcers, and no teeth problems. She reports arthralgia/joint pain (right knee) but reports no muscle aches, no muscle weakness, no back pain, and no swelling in the extremities. She reports frequent or severe headaches but reports no loss of consciousness, no weakness, no numbness, no seizures, no dizziness, and no tremor. She reports fatigue. She reports no fever, no night sweats, no significant weight gain, no significant weight loss, and no exercise intolerance. She reports no dry eyes, no vision change, and no irritation. She reports no difficulty hearing and no ear pain. She reports no chest pain, no arm pain on exertion, no shortness of breath when walking, no shortness of breath when lying down, no palpitations, and no known heart murmur. She reports no cough, no wheezing, no shortness of breath, no coughing up blood, and no sleep apnea. She reports no abdominal pain, no nausea, no vomiting, no constipation, normal appetite, no diarrhea, not vomiting blood, no dyspepsia, and no GERD. She reports no incontinence, no difficulty urinating, no hematuria, and no increased frequency. She reports no abnormal mole, no jaundice, no rashes, and no laceration. She reports no depression, no sleep disturbances, feeling safe in a relationship, no alcohol abuse, no anxiety, no hallucinations, and no suicidal thoughts. She reports no swollen glands, no bruising, and no excessive bleeding. She reports no runny nose, no sinus pressure, no itching, no hives, and no frequent sneezing.

History—updated 04/05/2019

Breast cancer—stable, sees oncology, on tamoxifen for 2

years

Depressive disorder—major, partially managed on SSRI

The provider should also be queried for E66.2 Morbid (severe) obesity with alveolar hypoventilation. The **body mass index (BMI)** is noted to be 36.6 on the DOS and the patient has comorbidities of hypertension, hyperlipidemia, and obstructive **sleep apnea (OSA)**.

This note validates that the **breast cancer** is an active problem which is being treated. The provider documented that the patient is undergoing treatment with tamoxifen and is seeing an oncology provider. The history portion of this note also shows that it was updated on the date of service (DOS).

Physical Exam

Patient is a 54-year-old female.

Constitutional

General Appearance: well-developed, appears stated age, and obese.

Level of Distress: comfortable.

Psychiatric

Mental Status: alert and normal affect.

Orientation: oriented to time, place, and person. Insight: good judgment.

Cardiovascular

Precordial Exam: no heaves or precordial thrills and non-displaced focal PMI. Rate And Rhythm: regular.

Heart Sounds: no rub, gallop, or click and normal S1 and physiologically split S2.

Systolic Murmur: not heard.

Diastolic Murmur: not heard

Extremities

No cyanosis, edema, or peripheral signs of emboli

Neurologic

Motor: tremor of neck and face and arms

A/P

1. Mixed hyperlipidemia—continue meds
2. Benign essential hypertension—continue meds
3. Insomnia—discussed sleep hygiene/caffeine curfew
4. Anxiety/depression—continue meds/consider seeing psych
5. Obesity—discussed increasing activity and decreasing caloric intake

It is necessary to query the provider for additional information about the **depression**. There is insufficient documentation to code major **depressive** disorder.

HCC Category	ICD-10-CM Code Description	RAF Value	Validated by Current Documentation	Improved Documentation
HCC 58	F33.41 Major depressive disorder, recurrent, in partial remission	0.395	No	Yes
HCC 12	C50.919 Malignant neoplasm of unspecified site of unspecified female breast	0.146	Yes	Yes
HCC 22	E66.2 Obesity hypoventilation syndrome (OHS)	0.273	No	Yes
Demographics	54-year-old, female, not Medicaid eligible	0.263	Yes	Yes
Total RAF			0.409	1.077

Coding Scenario 2

Result type: History and Physical Note	**Performed By/Author:** Doe MD, John on January 11, 2019
Result date: January 11, 2019	**Verified By:** Doe MD, John on January 11, 2019
Result status: Auth (Verified)	**Encounter info:** (IPE) Emergency - IP, 1/11/2019 - 1/12/2019
Result Title/Subject: History and Physical	

* Final Report *

History and Physical

Patient: Paul Doe	**Age:** 91 years	**Sex:** Male
Associated Diagnoses: None	**DOB:** 12/27/1936	

Chief Complaint: slurred speech, facial droop, fall **Author:** Black, MD Brian

History of Present Illness

91 yo M PMH significant for A-fib not on anticoagulation, HTN, asthma, colon CA s/p resection 2 years prior who is BIBAf for acute onset of slurred speech, left lower facial droop following fall. Patient and wife note around 830 PM last night, he sustained a slow fall in his home. He is unsure if he lost balance but had difficulty standing back up on his own but was able to be seated into chair by his wife. He then noticed that he had a difficult time speaking and his wife noted he had a left lower facial droop. She suspected he has having a stroke and gave him approximately 250 mg of Aspirin. Wife then called EMS, and patient and wife both note that his symptoms were improving already in the ambulance. Symptoms were essentially resolved by the time he arrived to the ED here, which was approximately 30 mins after onset of symptoms. He had otherwise been feeling well except for a mild cough which started about 10 days ago and has mostly resolved. He notes he was given a cough suppressant with bactrim by PCP, which he has since completed. He otherwise denies any fevers, chills, dizziness, shortness of breath, chest pain, palpitations, nausea/vomiting, bowel changes, urinary changes, blood in stool.

Review of Systems

12 point ROS reviewed and negative except as above

Past Medical History

as noted above.

Allergies (1) Active Reaction: quiNIDine Affect his liver

Social History

denies tobacco, quit in 1986

denies etoh or drug use

Family History

mother- colon CA

Brother- throat CA

Home Medications (6) Active

atenolol 25 mg oral tablet See Instructions

finasteride 5 mg oral tablet 5 mg = 1 tab, PO, daily

loratadine 10 mg, PO, daily

multivitamin 1 cap, PO, daily

tamsulosin 0.4 mg oral capsule 0.4 mg = 1 cap, PO, daily

Unlisted Med See Instructions

Current Vitals (past 48hrs, max 5 results)

Dt/Tm	Temp	BP	MAP	Pulse	RR	SpO2	FiO2	O2 Therapy
01/11/18 00:30	-----	122/60	81	88	18	96%	-----	Room air
01/11/18 00:11	-----	129/58	82	78	18	96%	-----	Room air
01/10/18 22:45	36.7	127/75	92	83	18	96%	-----	Room air

Tmax 24Hr: 36.7 DegC (98.1 DegF) 01/10/18 22:45 (Oral)

Tmax 36Hr: 36.7 DegC (98.1 DegF) 01/10/18 22:45 (Oral)

BMI: 17.44 (01/10/2018 23:10)

BMI is noted to be less than 19. The provider should be queried for malnutrition.

Physical Examination

General: Awake, alert, NAD

HEENT: Normo-cephalic, atraumatic; PERRL. Extraocular muscles are intact, sclera non-icteric

Neck: Trachea midline

Lungs: Clear to auscultation bilaterally

Cardiac: Irregular rate/rhythm, S1 and S2 with no murmurs

Abdomen: Soft, non-tender and non-distended with good bowel sounds

Extremities: No cyanosis or edema

Skin: No rashes or lesion

Neurological: Cranial nerves II through XII grossly intact, motor- 5/5 throughout large muscle groups, sensation-intact throughout, cerebellar- finger to nose wnl, alert and oriented to person, place and time

Psychiatric Evaluation: Normal mood and affect, normal judgement and insight

All Results (36 Hrs)

All labs personally reviewed.

Radiology Results (Past 36 Hours)

CT Head w/o Contrast STROKE CO   Performed By/Author: Dr. Moore, MD Sandra M

IMPRESSION: Subtle hyper-intensity within an insular branch of the left middle cerebral artery may reflect vessel occlusion or atherosclerotic calcification. Recommend CTA head. No acute intracranial hemorrhage is appreciated. No definite acute parenchymal changes are identified. Probable old left basal ganglia infarct. These findings were discussed with Dr. Moore, MD

XR Hip 2 View Left + Pelvis   Performed By/Author: Dr. Moore, MD Sandra M

IMPRESSION: No acute abnormality.

XR Chest 1 View   Performed By/Author: Dr. Moore, MD Sandra M

IMPRESSION: Multifocal airspace opacities suspicious for pneumonia. Recommend follow-up to resolution.

CTA Head/Neck w/ Con STROKE CO   Performed By/Author: Dr. Moore, MD Sandra M

IMPRESSION: Focal complete occlusion of a left middle cerebral artery M2 insular branch. Findings correspond to the dense artery on the non-contrast head CT. 50% right ICA stenosis and 60% left ICA stenosis in the neck. Patchy upper lobe airspace opacities suggestive of multifocal pneumonia. These findings were discussed with Dr. Moore, MD Sandra M

ASSESSMENT / PLAN

91 yo M PMH significant for A-fib not on anticoagulation, HTN, asthma, colon CA s/p resection 15 years prior who is BIBA from for acute onset of slurred speech, left lower facial droop following fall.

1. TIA
    - symptoms resolved
    - CT head with old left basal ganglia infarct but no acute findings
    - CTA head/neck w/ focal complete occlusion of left MCA M2 insular branch, 60% left ICA stenosis, 50% right ICA stenosis
    - Neurology consulted in ED- appreciate further recs
    - ASA, statin
    - check MRI brain
    - check 2d echo w/ bubble study
    - PT/OT eval
    - allow for permissive HTN first 24 hrs
2. Permanent atrial fibrillation- rate controlled
    - not on anticoagulation, dx in late 1980s and has not been on anticoagulation since for > 25 years
    - CHADS2vasc score of 5 and would likely be candidate for anticoagulation if bleeding risk not significantly elevated
    - will defer timing of anticoagulation to neurology, await MRI results
3. Multifocal PNA- largely asymptomatic
    - incidentally noted on CXR, CTA neck
    - reports recent tx w/ bactrim
    - possibly remnant of recent PNA, however given leukocytosis, imaging findings and tx w/ only bactrim recently, will tx
    - ceftriaxone/doxy
    - f/u sputum cx, pna serologies
4. HTN
    - allow permissive HTN up to SBP 220 first 24 hrs
    - hold atenolol
5. Chronic asthma
    - no exacerbation > 70 years per patient
    - uses inhalers bid, prn
6. hx colon CA s/p resection 2 years ago
    - pt reports taking vitamins and holistic cures
    - Oncology recs appreciated

It is necessary to query the provider for additional information about the chronic asthma. There is insufficient documentation to code **COPD.**

16

HCC Category	ICD-10-CM Code Description	RAF Value	Validated by Current Documentation	Improved Documentation
HCC 58	G45.9-Transient cerebral ischemic attack, unspecified	0.330	Yes	Yes
HCC 18	I48.2- Chronic atrial fibrillation	0.368	Yes	Yes
HCC 21	E46-Unspecified protein-calorie malnutrition	0.713	No	Yes
HCC 11	C18.9-Malignant neoplasm of colon, unspecified	0.317	Yes	Yes
HCC 111	J44.9 - Chronic obstructive pulmonary disease, unspecified	0.346	No	Yes
Demographics	91-year-old, male, Medicaid eligible	0.848 + 0.177	Yes	Yes
Total RAF			2.040	3.039

There is an additional RAF value added for the Medicaid eligibility which adds 0.177 to this patient's risk adjustment factor.

ALCOHOL ABUSE VERSUS DEPENDENCE

In the fifth edition of the Diagnostic and Statistical Manual of Mental Disorders (DSM-5), the American Society of Addiction Medicine created a category called ***"Substance Use Disorders."*** This category combines the concepts of *"substance abuse"* and *"substance dependence"* into a single disorder, measured on a continuum from mild to severe.

A. Diagnostic Criteria for Substance Use Disorders

DSM-5 defines substance use disorder as a problematic pattern of substance use leading to clinically significant impairment or distress, as manifested by *at least two* of the following occurring in a 12-month period:

DSM-5 Criteria for Substance Use Disorders

1. Substance is often taken in larger amounts or over a longer period of time than was intended
2. Persistent desire or unsuccessful efforts to cut down or control substance use
3. Great deal of time spent in activities to obtain the substance, use the substance, or recover from its effects
4. Craving or strong desire to use the substance
5. Recurrent use resulting in failure to fulfill major role obligations at work, school, home
6. Continued substance use despite persistent or recurrent social or interpersonal problems
7. Important social, occupational, or recreational activities are given up or reduced because of substance use
8. Recurrent substance use in situations in which it is physically hazardous
9. Substance use is continued despite knowledge of having a persistent or recurrent physical or psychological problem that is likely to have been caused or exacerbated by the substance

10. Tolerance, as defined by either of the following:

    a. A need for markedly increased amounts of the substance to achieve desired effect

    b. A markedly diminished effect with continued use of the same amount of substance

11. Withdrawal, as manifested by either of the following:

    a. Characteristic withdrawal syndrome for the substance

    b. Use of the substance or closely related substance is taken to relieve or avoid withdrawal symptoms

Note: Symptoms of **tolerance and withdrawal** occurring in the context of appropriate medical treatment with prescribed medications (e.g., opioid analgesics, sedatives, stimulants) are specifically **not counted** when diagnosing a substance use disorder. Furthermore, the DSM states:

> *"The appearance of normal, expected pharmacological tolerance and withdrawal during the course of medical treatment has been known to lead to an erroneous diagnosis of "addiction," even when these were the only symptoms present."*

B. Severity of Substance Use Disorders

1. Mild: Presence of 2-3 symptoms

2. Moderate: Presence of 4-5 symptoms

3. Severe: Presence of 6 or more symptoms

C. Remission, Controlled Environment, & Maintenance Therapy

Remission occurs when an individual with the disorder has met *none* of the criteria for substance use disorder (except craving) for at least three months. Remission is divided into:

❖ **Early remission:** ≥3 to <12 months without meeting substance use disorders criteria

(except craving)

❖ **Sustained remission:** ≥12 months without meeting substance use disorders criteria (except craving) Remission can be further specified as:

    ❖ **"In a controlled environment"** – When the individual in remission is in a supervised residential setting where access to alcohol and controlled substances is restricted

"On maintenance therapy" – When the individual in remission is being maintained on a prescribed medication (e.g., agonist, partial agonist, agonist/antagonist, or full antagonist)

D. Substance Use Disorders & ICD-10

Unlike DSM-5, ICD-10-CM continues to employ the concepts of *"substance abuse"* and *"substance dependence."*

Substance abuse represents a maladaptive pattern of drug-taking, which may include detriments to social functioning, to physical well-being and/or to mental health in patients who have not yet reached a state of physical dependence.

Substance dependence is defined as a chronic mental and physical condition related to the patient's pattern of drug-taking that is characterized by behavioral and physiological responses, which may include:

➤ A compulsion to take the drug in order to experience its psychic effects, or to avoid the discomfort of its absence

➤ An inability to stop the use of the drug despite strong incentives

    Physical dependence (i.e., tolerance and withdrawal)

Documentation Guidance

When documenting substance use disorders, include the following:

✓ Severity – mild, moderate, etc.

✓ Pattern of use – continuous use, in remission, relapsed, etc.

✓ Substance-induced mood/psychotic symptoms – depression, hallucinations, anxiety, etc.

✓ Current presentation – intoxication, drunkenness, withdrawal

✓ Treatment plan – rehabilitation, maintenance therapy (specify drug), AA, etc.

Coding Guidance

- *Substance use disorders* – The "substance use disorders" of DSM-5 are reported in ICD-10 as follows:

DSM-5 Diagnosis		***ICD-10 Category***
Substance use disorder, mild	→	Substance abuse
Substance use disorder, moderate	→	Substance dependence
Substance use disorder, severe	→	Substance dependence

- *Substance use, abuse, and dependence* – When use, abuse and dependence of the same substance are documented in the encounter note, only one code should be assigned based on the following hierarchy:

If...		***Then report...***
Both use and abuse are documented	→	Abuse
Both abuse and dependence are documented	→	Dependence
Use, abuse and dependence are documented	→	Dependence
Both use and dependence are documented	→	Dependence

- *Drug dependence in context of appropriate medical treatment* – Physical dependence (i.e., tolerance and withdrawal) can develop with the chronic use of many drugs: this can include prescription drugs, even if taken as instructed. ICD-10-CM does not distinguish between this normal, expected response and other forms of drug dependence. Any type of drug dependency (i.e., prescribed, non-prescribed [illicit], physiological and/or behavioral) is coded similarly.

Clinical overview

Definition

Atrial fibrillation is an arrhythmia (an abnormal rhythm of the heart) in which the two small upper chambers of the heart, called the atria, "fibrillate" (contract very fast and irregularly) and quiver instead of beating effectively.

Background

Atrial fibrillation is the most common type of heart arrhythmia. When the atria of the heart quiver or fibrillate, blood is not pumped completely out of the atria; thus, blood may pool and clot. If a blood clot is pumped out of the heart, it can lodge in an artery in the brain and block blood flow, causing a stroke. Further, atrial fibrillation that is not controlled can weaken the heart, causing heart failure (a condition in which the heart cannot effectively pump blood to the body).

Types

- **Paroxysmal:** Atrial fibrillation begins suddenly and stops on its own. Symptoms range from mild to severe; can last seconds, minutes, hours or days; and can occur intermittently.
- **Persistent:** Atrial fibrillation persists and continues until it is resolved with treatment.
- **Permanent:** Atrial fibrillation cannot be stopped with the usual treatment. Paroxysmal and persistent atrial fibrillation both can lead to permanent atrial fibrillation.

Possible causes

- High blood pressure
- Heart attacks
- Abnormal heart valves
- Congenital heart defects
- Metabolic imbalances, such as an overactive thyroid
- Stimulants, such as medications, caffeine, tobacco or alcohol
- Emphysema or other lung diseases
- Prior heart surgeries
- Viral infections
- Stress related to surgery or other illnesses
- Sleep apnea

Note: Sometimes the cause is not known.

Signs and symptoms

- Palpitations (sensations of a racing, irregular heartbeat or a pounding or flopping in the chest)
- Decreased blood pressure
- Weakness or fatigue
- Lightheadedness
- Confusion
- Shortness of breath
- Chest pain

Note: In some cases, there may be no symptoms.

Diagnostic tools

- Medical history and physical exam
- Electrocardiogram (ECG or EKG)
- Holter monitor
- Cardiac event recording
- Echocardiogram
- Blood tests (to check for metabolic problems or substances in the blood that can cause atrial fibrillation)
- Chest X-ray (to monitor for complications, such as fluid buildup in the lungs, or to check for other conditions that may be responsible for signs and symptoms)

Treatment

- Blood-thinning medications to prevent clots
- Medications to control the heart rate and rhythm
- Medical procedures, such as electrical cardioversion (electrical shock delivered to reset the heart rhythm) or ablation therapy that destroys tiny areas of heart tissue that are causing atrial fibrillation by firing off abnormal electrical impulses (radiofrequency ablation, destruction by electrical current; or cryoablation, destruction by extreme cold energy)
- Pacemaker implantation
- Surgical procedures called Maze procedures that create a pattern of scar tissue in the heart (Since scar tissue does not conduct electricity, the abnormal electrical impulses causing the problem are disrupted.)

Documentation tips for physicians

Abbreviations
A good rule of thumb for any medical record is to limit – or avoid altogether – the use of acronyms and abbreviations. While AF is a commonly accepted medical abbreviation for atrial fibrillation, this abbreviation has other meanings (example: atrial flutter). The meaning of an abbreviation or acronym can often be determined based on context, but this is not always true. Best practice is to always document atrial fibrillation by spelling it out in full.

Subjective
- The subjective section of the office note should show the patient was screened for current symptoms related to atrial fibrillation.

Objective
- The objective section should include any current associated physical exam findings (such as "irregularly irregular" rhythm or increased heart rate) and related diagnostic testing results.
- If there are no current related exam findings, the objective section should show the patient was evaluated for related findings.

Current atrial fibrillation
- Do not use the descriptor "history of" to describe current atrial fibrillation. In diagnosis coding, the descriptor "history of" implies the condition occurred in the past and is no longer a current problem.

Historical atrial fibrillation
- Temporary or transient atrial fibrillation that occurred in the past and is no longer present should not be documented as if it is current.
- This is true even in the presence of ongoing, chronic anticoagulation therapy that is being used in case a historical atrial fibrillation should ever recur.

Medications
- Clearly link atrial fibrillation to any medication specifically being used in the treatment of atrial fibrillation.
- Include the purpose of each medication, for example: antiarrhythmic to control heart rate and rhythm, anticoagulant to prevent blood clots.

Final assessment/impression
- Document current atrial fibrillation to the highest level of specificity, using all applicable descriptors (paroxysmal, persistent, chronic, permanent).
- Document the current status of atrial fibrillation (stable, worsening, controlled with medication, etc.).

Plan
- Document a specific and concise treatment plan for atrial fibrillation.
  - Example: "Continue amiodarone for atrial fibrillation and follow-up in 3 months."

Documentation and coding examples

Example 1	
Final diagnosis	Paroxysmal atrial fibrillation
ICD-10-CM code	I48.0

Example 2	
Final diagnosis	Persistent atrial fibrillation
ICD-10-CM code	I48.1

Example 3	
Final diagnosis	Chronic atrial fibrillation
ICD-10-CM code	I48.2

Example 4	
Final diagnosis	Permanent atrial fibrillation
ICD-10-CM code	I48.2

Example 5	
Final diagnosis	Unspecified atrial fibrillation
ICD-10-CM code	I48.91

Example 6	
Final diagnosis	History of atrial fibrillation, on prophylactic anticoagulation with warfarin
ICD-10-CM codes	Z86.79 Personal history of other diseases of the circulatory system Z79.01 Long term (current) use of anticoagulant

ICD-10-CM tips and resources for coders

Current atrial fibrillation

According to the ICD-10-CM manual, current atrial fibrillation classifies to the following codes:

Alphabetic index

Fibrillation

atrial or auricular (established) I48.91

chronic I48.2

paroxysmal I48.Ø

permanent I48.2

persistent I48.1

TABULAR LIST

I48.Ø   Paroxysmal atrial fibrillation

I48.1   Persistent atrial fibrillation

I48.2   Chronic atrial fibrillation
    (Includes permanent atrial fibrillation)

I48.91 Unspecified atrial fibrillation

History of atrial fibrillation

No history code is available specifically for "personal history of atrial fibrillation" or "personal history of cardiac arrhythmia."

- The best code available is Z86.79, personal history of other diseases of the circulatory system.

Atrial fibrillation and anticoagulation therapy

Code Z79.Ø1 represents long-term (current) use of anticoagulants.

Background

The quivering and ineffective beating of the heart that occur with atrial fibrillation can cause blood to pool in the heart chambers, resulting in clots inside the heart.

If the heart spontaneously returns to a normal rhythm and suddenly starts pumping blood effectively, a blood clot can be dislodged and pumped out of the heart and to an artery in the brain. The blood clot can ultimately lodge in the brain artery, blocking blood flow with vital oxygen and nutrients to that area of the brain. This is known as an ischemic stroke and can lead to devastating neurological deficits, disability or even death.

To prevent this potential complication, blood-thinning drugs (anticoagulants), such as Coumadin (warfarin), are used to prevent the development of blood clots inside the heart.

Atrial fibrillation and anticoagulant therapy – continued

Key points:

- Unlike antiarrhythmic drugs, anticoagulation therapy does not treat or control the atrial fibrillation arrhythmia itself. Rather, anticoagulants are used to prevent the complication of blood clot formation in the heart as previously described.

- A coder cannot assume anticoagulation therapy is being used to treat atrial fibrillation when there is no documented link between the two in the record.

- Even when the medical record links anticoagulation therapy to the treatment of atrial fibrillation, this does not necessarily mean atrial fibrillation is current, since long-term anticoagulant therapy (Z79.Ø1) may be used to:

    a) Prevent blood clots in a patient with **current** atrial fibrillation (category I48);

                    OR

    b) Prevent blood clots in a patient with a past history of atrial fibrillation (Z86.79) in case atrial fibrillation should ever recur.

Ultimately, code assignment is based on the physician's specific description of atrial fibrillation in the individual medical record, i.e., whether the medical record describes and supports atrial fibrillation as current versus historical.

Postoperative atrial fibrillation

Postoperative atrial fibrillation with no further description classifies to the following codes:

- I97.89   Other postprocedural complications and disorders of the circulatory system, not elsewhere classified

- I48.91   Unspecified atrial fibrillation

References: American Heart Association; ICD-10-CM Official Guidelines for Coding and Reporting; Mayo Clinic; National Heart, Lung and Blood Institute; WebMD

Documentation tips for physicians

Breast cancer site(s) – primary and secondary

Document whether current breast cancer is primary, secondary or in situ. Also document:

- Laterality (right or left)
- The specific site of primary cancer, including the location within the breast (areola, nipple, upper outer quadrant, central portion, etc.)
- The specific secondary site(s)

Current versus historical breast cancer

- Do not use the phrase "history of" to describe a current primary breast cancer. In diagnosis coding, "history of" means the condition is historical and no longer exists as a current problem.
- In the final impression, do not document a simple statement of "breast cancer" to describe a historical primary breast cancer that was previously excised or eradicated and for which there is:
  a) No active treatment; and
  b) No evidence of disease or recurrence.
  In this scenario, it is appropriate to document "history of breast cancer," along with details of past diagnosis and treatment.

Treatment plan

- Document a clear and concise plan of care.
- Clearly indicate whether current therapy represents:
  o Active treatment of current breast cancer; versus
  o Surveillance of a historical breast cancer to monitor for recurrence.
- When adjuvant therapy is used, clearly state its purpose (whether the goal of adjuvant therapy is curative, palliative or preventive*).
- If referrals are made or consultations requested, indicate to whom or where the referral is made or from whom consultation advice is requested.
- Document when the patient is to be seen again.

*Adjuvant therapy for breast cancer

Adjuvant treatment is additional treatment given after the primary treatment has been completed to:
a) Destroy any remaining cancer cells that may be undetectable, and/or
b) Lower the risk that the cancer will come back.

Adjuvant therapy – continued

Adjuvant treatment may include chemotherapy, radiation therapy, hormone therapy, targeted therapy or biological therapy. Examples of drugs used as adjuvant therapy for breast cancer include Tamoxifen, Arimidex, Faslodex and Femara.

Document the purpose of adjuvant treatment of breast cancer in each individual case, i.e., whether it is:

- Curative – given to cure breast cancer
- Palliative – given to relieve the symptoms and reduce the suffering caused by breast cancer without effecting a cure.
- Prophylactic/preventive – given to keep breast cancer from recurring in a person who has already been treated for breast cancer

ICD-10-CM tips and resources for coders

Category C5Ø, malignant neoplasm of breast

- **Includes:** connective tissue of the breast; Paget's disease of the breast; Paget's disease of the nipple
- **Excludes1**: skin of the breast (C44.5Ø1, C44.511, C44.521, C44.591)
- Use an additional code to identify estrogen receptor status (Z17.Ø, Z17.1).
- Fifth and sixth characters are required to specify location, gender and laterality.

Coding the breast cancer site

Always code breast cancer with the highest level of specificity. Carefully review the medical record documentation, noting the particular site of cancer within the breast.

Sometimes physicians and other health care providers describe the site of breast cancer as positions on a clock. In those cases, the following illustrations of breast cancer quadrants and "clock" positions can be used to assist in code selection.

Breast cancer quadrants and "clock" positions

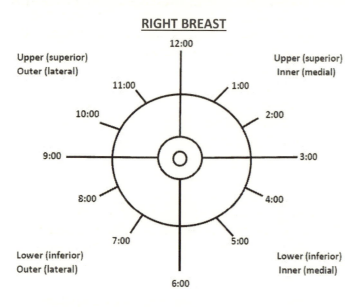

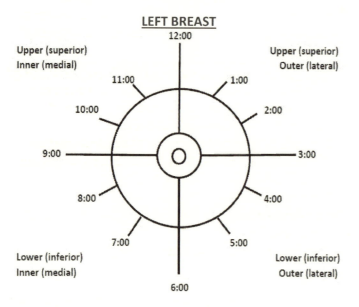

Malignant neoplasm of overlapping sites within the breast classifies to subcategory C5Ø.8- with fifth and sixth characters to specify gender and laterality. Subcategory C5Ø.8 includes (but is not limited to) the following:

      12:00   6:00
      3:00   9:00
      Midline of breast

Coding breast cancer as current

In general, code breast cancer as current when the medical record clearly documents active breast cancer that is receiving current active treatment (which in some cases may include adjuvant treatment in accordance with the guidelines noted on page 1)*; and/or when the record clearly shows breast cancer is still present but:

  a) It is unresponsive to treatment;
  b) The current treatment plan is observation only or "watchful waiting;" or
  c) The patient has refused further treatment.

Coding breast cancer as historical

Breast cancer is coded as historical (Z85.3) after the breast cancer has been excised or eradicated, there is no active treatment directed to the breast cancer and there is currently no evidence of disease or recurrence.

Encounter for follow-up examination after treatment for malignant neoplasm has been completed is coded as ZØ8. This code includes medical surveillance following completed treatment (i.e., monitoring for cancer recurrence) and *Excludes1* aftercare following medical care (Z43 – Z49, Z51). Code ZØ8 advises to use an additional code to identify any acquired absence of organs (Z9Ø.-) and personal history of malignant neoplasm (Z85.-).

References: ICD-10-CM Official Guidelines for Coding and Reporting; Mayo Clinic; MedlinePlus; National Cancer Institute

Clinical overview

Definition

Cardiomyopathy is a disease of the heart muscle that impairs the function of the heart.

Types

Cardiomyopathy can be classified as primary or secondary and ischemic or nonischemic.

- **Primary cardiomyopathy** is a noninflammatory disease of the heart muscle, often of obscure or unknown cause, that occurs in the absence of other cardiac conditions or systemic disease processes.
- **Secondary cardiomyopathy** is caused by a known medical condition (such as hypertension, valve disease, congenital heart disease or coronary artery disease).
- **Ischemic cardiomyopathy** is caused by coronary artery disease and heart attacks, which result in lack of blood flow to the heart muscle, thereby causing damage to the heart muscle.
- **Nonischemic cardiomyopathy** is a type of cardiomyopathy not related to coronary artery disease or poor coronary artery blood flow. There are three main types of nonischemic cardiomyopathy:
  - **Dilated cardiomyopathy (also known as congestive cardiomyopathy)** – This is the most common type of cardiomyopathy. In this disorder, the heart's main pumping chamber – the left ventricle – becomes enlarged (dilated), its pumping ability becomes less forceful and blood doesn't flow as easily through the heart.
  - **Hypertrophic cardiomyopathy** – This type involves abnormal growth or thickening of the heart muscle, particularly affecting the muscle of the left ventricle. As thickening occurs, the heart tends to stiffen and the size of the pumping chamber may shrink, interfering with the heart's ability to deliver blood to the body.
  - **Restrictive cardiomyopathy** – The heart muscle in people with restrictive cardiomyopathy becomes rigid and less elastic, meaning the heart can't properly expand and fill with blood between heartbeats.

Some cardiomyopathies can be reversible. For example:
- Alcoholic cardiomyopathy sometimes can be reversed with complete cessation of alcohol intake.
- Takotsubo cardiomyopathy is a reversible, stress-induced cardiomyopathy.

Causes

The cause is usually unknown (primary cardiomyopathy), although contributing factors sometimes can be identified. Some of the possible known causes include:

- Long-term high blood pressure
- Coronary artery disease
- Heart valve problems
- Chronic rapid heart rate
- Certain viral infections
- Some chemotherapy drugs
- Pregnancy
- Excessive, long-term use of alcohol
- Heart damage, due to a previous heart attack
- Metabolic disorders (thyroid disease, diabetes, etc.)
- Nutritional deficiencies of essential vitamins and minerals
- Abuse of cocaine or antidepressant medications
- Hemochromatosis – disorder where iron is not properly metabolized, causing build-up in various organs, including heart muscle (This can lead to a weakening of the heart muscle, resulting in dilated cardiomyopathy.)

Signs and symptoms

There may be no signs or symptoms in the early stages of the disease. But as the condition advances, signs and symptoms usually appear and may include:
- Shortness of breath, especially with physical exertion
- Swelling of lower extremities, abdomen and neck veins
- Fatigue
- Chest pain
- Irregular heartbeats
- Heart murmurs
- Dizziness and lightheadedness
- Fainting

Possible complications

- Heart failure
- Blood clots
- Heart valve problems with associated murmurs
- Cardiac arrest and sudden death

Diagnostic tools

- Medical history and physical exam
- Blood tests, such as measurement of brain natriuretic peptide (BNP), a protein produced in the heart (The

Clinical overview

Diagnostic tools – continued

blood level of BNP increases when the heart is under stress from heart failure, a common complication of cardiomyopathy.)

- Chest X-ray (to check for signs such as enlarged heart or fluid buildup in lungs)
- Electrocardiogram (ECG or EKG)
- Holter and cardiac event monitoring
- Echocardiogram
- Cardiac stress testing
- Cardiac magnetic resonance imaging (MRI)
- Cardiac catheterization and heart biopsy

Treatment

- Lifestyle changes:
  - Heart-healthy diet
  - Weight control
  - Stress management
  - Physical activity and exercise
  - Smoking cessation
- Medications:
  - Blood thinners to prevent clots
  - Antiarrhythmics to control heart rate and rhythm
  - Antihypertensives for blood pressure control
  - Diuretics ("water pills") to remove excess sodium and reduce excess fluid in the blood
- Nonsurgical procedure:
  - Alcohol septal ablation, in which a type of alcohol (ethanol) is injected through a tube into the small artery that supplies blood to the thickened area of heart muscle. The alcohol shrinks the thickened heart tissue to a more normal size, allowing blood to flow freely through the ventricle of the heart, which results in improved symptoms.
- Cardiac device implantation:
  - Pacemaker
  - Cardioverter-defibrillator
  - Left ventricular assist device
- Surgical procedures:
  - Heart transplant (a last resort for severe, end-stage cardiomyopathy that cannot be controlled by other means)

Documentation tips for physicians

Abbreviations

A good rule of thumb for any medical record is to limit – or avoid altogether – the use of abbreviations. There are several commonly used medical abbreviations for the different types of cardiomyopathy (CM, CMP, HCM, HOCM, etc.), but some of these abbreviations have other meanings. The meaning of an abbreviation can often be determined based on context, but this is not always true. Best practice is to always document the specific type of cardiomyopathy by spelling it out in full.

Subjective

- The subjective section of the office note should show the patient was screened for current complaints or symptoms related to cardiomyopathy.

Objective

- The objective section of the office note should include any current associated physical exam findings (such as edema/swelling of the lower extremities, abdomen or neck veins) and related diagnostic testing results.
- If there are no current related exam findings, the objective section should show the patient was evaluated for related findings.

Current cardiomyopathy

- Do not use the descriptor "history of" to describe current cardiomyopathy. In diagnosis coding, "history of" means the condition occurred in the past and is no longer a current problem.

Historical/transient cardiomyopathy

- Temporary or transient cardiomyopathy that occurred in the past and is no longer present should not be documented as if it is current.

Final assessment/impression

- The term "cardiomyopathy" is broad and nonspecific; therefore, it is imperative to describe the particular type of cardiomyopathy to the highest level of specificity.
- Clearly link secondary cardiomyopathy to the underlying causative condition by using terms such as "due to," "secondary to," "associated with," "related to," etc.
- Document the current status of cardiomyopathy (stable, improved, worsening, etc.).

Plan

- Document a specific and concise treatment plan for cardiomyopathy.
  - Example: "Continue current cardiac medications and keep appointment next month for annual evaluation with Cardiovascular Associates."

Documentation and coding examples

Example 1	
Final diagnosis	Cardiomyopathy (nonspecific)
ICD-10-CM code	I42.9 (unspecified code)

Example 2	
Final diagnosis	Ischemic dilated cardiomyopathy
ICD-10-CM code	I25.5

Example 3	
Final diagnosis	Hypertensive cardiomyopathy
ICD-10-CM code	I11.9, I43

Example 4	
Final diagnosis	Cardiomyopathy due to sarcoidosis
ICD-10-CM code	D86.85

Example 5	
Final diagnosis	Metabolic cardiomyopathy
ICD-10-CM codes	E88.9, I43

Example 6	
Final diagnosis	Restrictive cardiomyopathy
ICD-10-CM code	I42.5

Example 7	
Final diagnosis	Rheumatic cardiomyopathy
ICD-10-CM code	I09.0

Example 8	
Final diagnosis	End-stage dilated cardiomyopathy
ICD-10-CM code	I42.0

ICD-10-CM tips and resources for coders

Basics of coding cardiomyopathy

For accurate and specific diagnosis code assignment, the coder must:

a) Review the entire medical record to verify cardiomyopathy is current.

b) Note the exact cardiomyopathy description documented in the medical record; then, in accordance with ICD-10-CM official coding conventions and guidelines:

c) Search the alphabetic index for that specific description.

d) Verify the code in the tabular list, carefully following all instructional notes.

Many of the most common cardiomyopathies classify to category I42, cardiomyopathy.

- A fourth character is required to specify the particular type of cardiomyopathy.
- The broad and nonspecific final diagnosis of "cardiomyopathy" leads to the broad and nonspecific diagnosis code I42.9, cardiomyopathy, unspecified.
- Code I42.9 should be assigned only when no information in the medical record identifies the particular type of cardiomyopathy.

Hypertensive cardiomyopathy classifies to category I11, hypertensive heart disease, with an additional code of I43, cardiomyopathy in diseases classified elsewhere.

Congestive cardiomyopathy is also known as dilated cardiomyopathy. Both of these descriptions classify to code I42.Ø, dilated cardiomyopathy.

- Congestive cardiomyopathy often is associated with congestive heart failure and basically has the same symptoms. Treatment typically focuses on management of the congestive heart failure; therefore, heart failure (I5Ø.-) is reported as the principal diagnosis with an additional code for the cardiomyopathy.

Hypertrophic cardiomyopathy can be obstructive or nonobstructive.

- I42.1 Obstructive hypertrophic cardiomyopathy
- I42.2 Other hypertrophic cardiomyopathy
  Includes nonobstructive hypertrophic cardiomyopathy

Reminders

- Use caution when coding cardiomyopathy from abbreviations (CM, HCM, HOCM, etc.). A code should not be assigned unless the meaning of the abbreviation is clear based on review of the entire medical record.
- Takotsubo cardiomyopathy is a reversible form of cardiomyopathy that classifies to code I51.81, Takotsubo syndrome. This code includes the following conditions:
  - Reversible left ventricular dysfunction following sudden emotional stress
  - Stress-induced cardiomyopathy
  - Takotsubo cardiomyopathy
  - Transient left ventricular ballooning syndrome
- Watch for modifying descriptors that affect code assignment (secondary, alcoholic, nutritional, metabolic or cardiomyopathy due to other diseases).
- Some secondary cardiomyopathies are coded with a single combination code, while other secondary cardiomyopathies require the use of two codes. See coding examples on page 3.
- The term "ischemic cardiomyopathy" is sometimes used to refer to a condition in which ischemic heart disease causes diffuse fibrosis or multiple infarction, leading to heart failure with left ventricular dilation. This is not a true cardiomyopathy; when no further clarification is available, this condition is coded to I25.5, ischemic cardiomyopathy.

References: American Hospital Association Coding Clinic; ICD-10-CM Official Guidelines for Coding and Reporting; ICD-10-CM and ICD-10-PCS Coding Handbook; Mayo Clinic; National Heart, Lung and Blood Institute

Clinical overview

Definition

A cerebrovascular accident, also known as a stroke, is an interruption or disruption of blood flow to the brain. When blood flow to an area of the brain stops, oxygen and nutrients cannot get to that area of the brain, and brain cells begin to die, resulting in permanent damage.

Types

- **Ischemic**: This type usually is caused by a blood clot that blocks a blood vessel (artery) that supplies oxygen-rich blood to the brain.
  - **Thrombotic stroke**: A blood clot forms inside an artery that supplies blood to the brain, blocking blood flow.
  - **Embolic stroke**: A blood clot forms in a vessel in another part of the body and then travels to and blocks a blood vessel in the brain.
  - **Other types of ischemic stroke** include very low blood pressure or narrowing or tears in the lining of one of the blood vessels that carry blood to the brain (i.e., carotid arteries), all of which decrease blood flow to the brain.
- **Hemorrhagic**: A blood vessel within the brain weakens and bursts, causing bleeding in the brain.
  - **Intracerebral hemorrhage**: Bleeding within the brain.
  - **Subarachnoid hemorrhage**: Bleeding into the space (subarachnoid space) between the inner layer and middle layer of the tissue covering the brain (the meninges).

Some causes of ischemic CVA

Conditions that can cause blood clots:
- Atherosclerosis (fatty substances in the blood collect on the walls of the arteries, causing narrowing of the vessel and slowing of blood flow, which can result in blood clot formation)
- Irregular heart rhythms, such as atrial fibrillation
- Certain drugs/medications
- Heart valve problems
- Congenital heart defects
- Blood-clotting disorders
- Inflammation or other disorders of blood vessels
- Injuries or surgeries involving blood vessels of the head or neck
- Cancer radiation treatments to the neck or brain

Some causes of hemorrhagic CVA

- Untreated or uncontrolled blood pressure
- Traumatic head and neck injuries
- Surgeries involving blood vessels of head and neck
- Blood-thinning medications
- Brain aneurysms (weak spots in walls of blood vessels in the brain) and other abnormalities of blood vessels in and around the brain
- Bleeding disorders
- Brain tumors
- Liver disease, which is associated with increased bleeding in general

Risk factors

- High blood pressure/hypertension
- Diabetes
- Obesity
- High cholesterol
- Cardiovascular disease
- Alcoholism
- Smoking
- Age (older than 55)
- Male gender
- Personal history of stroke
- Family history of stroke

Signs and symptoms

Sometimes there are no signs or symptoms. Signs or symptoms that may occur include, but are not limited to:
- Confusion, memory loss or impaired consciousness
- Change in personality, mood or emotions
- Headache
- Difficulty speaking or swallowing
- Loss of bowel or bladder function
- Loss of coordination or balance
- Difficulty walking
- Disturbances in vision, hearing or taste
- Unilateral paralysis, weakness or numbness

Complications

Complications depend on the type of stroke, degree of brain damage, the body systems affected and how quickly treatment is received. Complete recovery can occur, or there may be permanent residual deficits.

Clinical overview

Diagnostic tools

- Medical history and physical exam
- Laboratory blood testing (to check clotting factors, blood sugar and other blood chemicals)
- Electrocardiogram, echocardiogram and other cardiac monitoring to check for heart problems
- Ultrasound of the carotid arteries
- Computed tomography (CT) scan
- Magnetic resonance imaging (MRI)
- Magnetic resonance angiography (MRA) or CT angiography (CTA)

Treatment

An acute stroke represents a medical emergency. Prompt evaluation and treatment are critical to save brain tissue and avoid or reduce complications, residual effects and disability. Treatment depends on the cause and type of stroke and can include:

- For ischemic CVA, clot-busting drugs (must be administered within three hours of the onset of symptoms), blood thinners and carotid artery surgery, if indicated
- For hemorrhagic CVA, surgical intervention, if indicated to control bleeding
- Pain medications as indicated (e.g., for headache)
- Control and management of underlying causal conditions
- Physical, occupational and speech therapy for residual conditions

Documentation tips for physicians

Abbreviations

A good rule of thumb for any medical record is to limit – or avoid altogether – the use of abbreviations. While CVA is a commonly accepted medical abbreviation for cerebrovascular accident, best practice is as follows:

- The initial notation of an abbreviation or acronym should be spelled out in full with the abbreviation in parentheses: "Cerebrovascular accident (CVA)." Subsequent mention of the condition can be made using the acronym.
- The diagnosis should be spelled out in full in the final impression or plan.

Subjective

- The subjective section of the office note should document any current symptoms of cerebrovascular accident or patient complaints of any current residual deficits that are due to a past cerebrovascular accident.

Objective

- The objective section of the office note should include any current associated physical exam findings of current CVA or current residual deficits that are due to a past CVA.

Associated conditions and manifestations

- Clearly link associated conditions or manifestations to cerebrovascular accident by using linking terms such as "with," "due to," "secondary to," "associated with," "related to," etc. Examples:
  - "Acute ischemic CVA due to bilateral carotid artery atherosclerosis"
  - "Acute right ischemic CVA with associated left hemiplegia"
  - "Facial droop due to past hemorrhagic stroke that occurred six months ago"

Specificity

- Describe CVA, past or present, and any residual deficits with the highest level of specificity. For example:
  - Document the type of CVA (ischemic, hemorrhagic, postoperative, etc.), along with the cause, if known.
  - For related neurologic deficits, past or present, specify laterality (right or left, dominant or nondominant) or type (e.g., dysphagia oral phase, dysphagia pharyngeal phase, neurogenic dysphagia, etc.).

Current versus historical

- In the final assessment, do not document a past CVA as if it is current. An acute CVA represents a medical emergency that requires prompt medical treatment.
  - A final diagnosis stated simply "CVA" indicates a current CVA, which would not correlate with a treatment plan to "follow up in one year." Rather, this documentation suggests the CVA occurred in the past and should have been stated as "history of CVA."
- On the other hand, do not use past-tense terms such as "status post," "history of," "recent," "past," "prior," etc., to describe current residual deficits of past CVA.
  - In diagnosis coding, a residual deficit of CVA described as "history of," "status post," etc., indicates a historical condition that no longer exists as a current problem. Contrast these two examples:
    - **"History of CVA with facial weakness"** This documentation supports a historical condition (at some time in the past, the patient had a CVA with associated facial weakness).
    - **"Residual facial weakness due to past CVA"** This documentation supports current facial weakness due to past CVA.
  - Codes for residual effects/late effects/sequelae cannot be assigned based on the status of the condition in the past. Rather, code assignment must be based on documentation that clearly shows the residual condition is current. For example:
    - A final diagnosis of "residual left hemiparesis due to CVA one year ago" should be supported by a notation of left hemiparesis in the physical exam.

Treatment plan

Document a clear and concise treatment plan for CVA or residual deficits or disability related to past CVA. Examples:

- "Plan: Admit from emergency department to intensive care unit for acute cerebrovascular accident."
- "Referral to ABC provider for physical therapy evaluation and treatment of residual right-sided hemiparesis, due to past CVA."

ICD-10-CM tips and resources for coders

Coding basics

For accurate and specific diagnosis code assignment, the coder must:

a) Review the entire medical record to verify CVA or residual late effect of CVA is current.

b) Note the exact description of CVA or residual late effect of CVA that is documented in the medical record; then, in accordance with ICD-10-CM official coding conventions and guidelines:

1. Search the alphabetic index for that specific description.
2. Verify the code in the tabular list, carefully following all instructional notes.

Coding CVA and associated residual effects/sequelae

Categories	Description	Additional characters specify
I6Ø – I62	Nontraumatic intracranial hemorrhage	• Location • Affected artery • Laterality (right vs. left)
I63	Ischemic CVA due to thrombosis or embolus	• Cause (thrombosis, embolus or unspecified) • Location/affected artery • Laterality (right vs. left)
I69	Sequelae of CVA	• Type of CVA that caused the sequela • Specific sequela (residual late effect) • Laterality (right vs. left) with dominance or nondominance

Relevant terms

- Stenosis = narrowing
- Occlusion = complete or partial blockage
- Thrombus = blood clot that develops inside a blood vessel and stays in place
- Embolus = blood clot that develops inside a blood vessel but dislodges and travels to another location
- Cerebral arteries = arteries located inside the cerebrum of the brain. Examples:
  o Anterior cerebral artery, middle cerebral artery, posterior cerebral artery
- Precerebral arteries = arteries that lead to the cerebrum of the brain but are not located within the brain. Examples:
  o Vertebral artery, basilar artery, carotid artery

Current acute CVA

- The terms "stroke," "cerebral infarction" and "cerebrovascular accident" are often used interchangeably. These terms with no other specification or description are all indexed to the default code I63.9, cerebral infarction, unspecified.
  o Additional code(s) are assigned for any neurologic deficit associated with acute CVA, even when it has been resolved prior to discharge from the hospital.
- An acute CVA represents a medical emergency that requires prompt medical treatment. A final diagnosis of CVA with no supporting information and no related treatment plan does not support CVA as an acute event. Rather, this documentation suggests history of CVA. When there is no opportunity to query the physician for clarification, no diagnosis code can be assigned.
- Intraoperative or post-procedural CVA is coded when the medical record documentation clearly specifies cause-and-effect relationship between the medical intervention and the CVA. Proper code assignment depends on the specific descriptions documented in the record and the coding path in the ICD-10-CM coding manual.

Sequelae of CVA (formerly referred to as "late effects")

Codes from category I69, sequelae of cerebrovascular disease, include neurologic deficits that persist after the initial episode of care for CVA.

- The neurologic deficits caused by CVA may be present from the onset or may arise at any time after the onset of the CVA.
- When the patient is discharged from the initial episode of care for an acute CVA – even if transferred to a rehabilitation facility – any remaining residual neurologic deficit is considered a sequela/late effect and should be coded from category I69.
- Fourth characters specify the causal conditions as sequelae of:
  - I69.Ø-　Nontraumatic subarachnoid hemorrhage
  - I69.1-　Nontraumatic intracerebral hemorrhage
  - I69.2-　Other nontraumatic intracranial hemorrhage
  - I69.3-　Cerebral infarction

ICD-10-CM tips and resources for coders

Sequelae of CVA – continued

- Fifth characters specify the particular neurological deficits as follows:
    - Ø Unspecified sequelae
    - 1 Cognitive deficits
    - 2 Speech and language deficits
    - 3 Monoplegia of upper limb
    - 4 Monoplegia of lower limb
    - 5 Hemiplegia/hemiparesis
    - 6 Other paralytic syndrome
    - 9 Other sequelae

  Some codes have sixth characters for additional specificity, such as laterality, type, etc.
- Documentation must clearly link the residual deficit, late effect or sequela to the past CVA as the cause.
- In some cases, a patient is admitted with a current acute CVA with associated neurologic deficits, while at the same time having current residual neurologic deficits that result from an old, past or healed CVA. In this scenario, codes may be assigned together from categories I6Ø – I63 and I69 as indicated by the specific documentation in the medical record.
- Residual unilateral weakness related to past CVA is considered synonymous with hemiparesis and should be coded as such (AHA Coding Clinic guideline for residual right-sided weakness due to previous cerebral infarction, First Quarter 2015, Page 25).
- Residual weakness (without further description or specification and not described as unilateral) due to past CVA is coded as I69.398 and R53.1.
- Residual muscle weakness related to a past CVA is coded as I69.398 and M62.81.
- Codes from category I69, sequelae of cerebrovascular disease, that specify hemiplegia, hemiparesis and monoplegia identify whether the dominant or nondominant side is affected. If the affected side is documented but not specified as dominant or nondominant, and the classification system does not indicate a default, code selection is as follows:
    - o For ambidextrous patients, the default should be dominant.
    - o If the left side is affected, the default is nondominant.
    - o If the right side is affected, the default is dominant.

- When a neurological deficit related to past CVA is documented as "history of" or "status post" (as in "history of CVA with right hemiparesis"), it should not be coded as current if no supporting documentation shows the residual deficit is still present. Consider and contrast these two final diagnostic statements:
    - o **"History of CVA with right hemiparesis"**
      This description supports both CVA and right hemiparesis as historical – code as Z86.73.
    - o **"Residual right hemiparesis due to past CVA"**
      This description supports right hemiparesis as current and due to past CVA – code as I69.351.
- Codes for sequelae/residual late effects cannot be assigned based on the status of the condition in the past; rather, codes are assigned based on current status.
    - o Look for documentation in the medical record that clearly shows the residual neurological deficit that is a late effect or sequela of a past CVA is still present and current. For example, if the final diagnosis is "left hemiparesis due to past CVA," the physical exam should document left hemiparesis – or at the least, the physical exam should not contradict the final diagnosis (detailed musculoskeletal and neurologic exams with all normal findings would contradict the final diagnosis).
- Hemiparesis or hemiplegia documented without further specification or stated to be longstanding but of unspecified cause – i.e., no documented link to past CVA as the cause – is coded to category G81. Review and follow all instructional notes under this category.

History of CVA

History of CVA with no current associated residual deficits codes to Z86.73, personal history of transient ischemic attack (TIA), and cerebral infarction without residual deficits.

References: American Hospital Association Coding Clinic; ICD-10-CM Official Guidelines for Coding and Reporting; Mayo Clinic; MedlinePlus; Merck Manual; WebMD

Chronic Kidney Disease (CKD)   ICD-10-CM

Clinical overview

Definition

Chronic kidney disease (chronic renal failure) is longstanding, progressive deterioration of renal function.

Background

The kidneys maintain health by removing wastes and fluid from the body. The kidneys also perform these other important functions:

- Regulate body water and other chemicals in the blood, such as sodium, potassium, phosphorus and calcium
- Remove drugs and toxins
- Release hormones into the blood to regulate blood pressure, make red blood cells and promote strong bones

Causes

The main causes of CKD are hypertension and diabetes mellitus. Some of the other causes include:

- Glomerulonephritis – a group of diseases that cause inflammation and damage to the glomeruli (the filtering units of the kidney)
- Inherited diseases, such as polycystic kidney disease or sickle cell disease
- Congenital malformations (present at birth)
- Diseases of the immune system, such as lupus
- Obstructions caused by problems such as kidney stones, tumors or enlarged prostate gland in men
- Repeated urinary tract infections
- Lead poisoning
- Long-term use of medicines that damage the kidneys – for example, nonsteroidal anti-inflammatory drugs (NSAIDs), such as ibuprofen and naproxen

Note: Sometimes the cause is not known.

Signs and symptoms

There may be no symptoms in the early stages of CKD. As kidney function decreases, symptoms may include:

- Abnormal laboratory values (e.g., increased serum creatinine, blood urea nitrogen [BUN] or certain electrolytes)
- High blood pressure that is difficult to control
- Changes in urine output (e.g., urinating less or more frequently than normal)
- Swelling due to fluid buildup in the tissues (edema)

Signs and symptoms – continued

- Fatigue and weakness
- Loss of appetite
- Weight loss
- Nausea and/or vomiting
- Excessive sleepiness or inability to sleep
- Headaches
- Decreased mental sharpness, trouble concentrating
- Dry, itchy skin

Diagnostic tools

- Laboratory testing to check kidney function (urinalysis, blood testing for creatinine, urea, electrolytes, etc.)
- Glomerular filtration rate (GFR) – best test to measure level of kidney function and determine stage of kidney disease
- Imaging tests to evaluate for cause or type of CKD, including ultrasound, computed tomography (CT) scanning, magnetic resonance imaging (MRI)
- Renal biopsy (in some cases)

Treatment

Chronic kidney failure (disease) has no cure, but treatment can help control signs and symptoms, reduce complications and slow the progress of the disease. The first priority is controlling the condition responsible for the kidney failure and its complications (e.g., controlling diabetes or high blood pressure). Other treatments include:

- Proper diet (protein management along with salt, potassium and phosphorus restrictions may help slow disease progression)
- Daily exercise
- Avoidance of dehydration
- Avoidance of smoking and other tobacco products, alcohol and illegal drugs
- Avoidance of substances that are toxic to the kidneys, such as nonsteroidal anti-inflammatory drugs
- Treating complications

In end-stage kidney disease (when kidney function is reduced to 10-15 percent or less of capacity), conservative measures as outlined above are no longer enough. Dialysis or kidney transplant become the only options to support life.

Documentation tips for physicians

Abbreviations

A good rule of thumb for any medical record is to limit – or avoid altogether – the use of abbreviations. While CKD is a commonly accepted medical abbreviation for chronic kidney disease, best practice is as follows:

- The initial notation of an abbreviation should be spelled out in full with the abbreviation in parentheses: "chronic kidney disease (CKD)." Subsequent mention of the CKD can be made using the abbreviation.

Subjective

- In the subjective section of the office note, document the presence or absence of any current symptoms related to chronic kidney disease (e.g., fatigue, weakness, changes in urine output, etc.).

Objective

In the objective section of the office note, document:

- Any current associated physical exam finding (e.g., elevated blood pressure, edema, weight loss, etc.)
- Related diagnostic test results
- Presence of a surgically placed arteriovenous shunt for the purpose of dialysis, along with related exam findings (e.g., presence of a thrill or bruit)

Final assessment/impression

- Document the specific stage of chronic kidney disease. Remember that medical coders are not allowed to calculate the stage of CKD based on documentation of the GFR; the specific stage must be stated in the medical record.
- Include the current status of CKD (stable, worsening, improved, etc.).
- State the cause of CKD, if known. Use linking terms or descriptors that clearly show cause and effect (see "Chronic kidney disease and associated conditions" in the coding section on pages 3 and 4).

Treatment plan

- Document a specific, concise treatment plan for CKD.
- Include specific details of current dialysis status (hemodialysis, peritoneal dialysis, frequency, etc.).
- If referrals are made or consultations requested, the office note should indicate to whom or where the referral of consultation is made or from whom consultation advice is requested.

Treatment plan – continued

Document when the patient will be seen again, even if only on an as-needed basis.

Associated conditions

When no other cause is specified, ICD-10-CM presumes a cause-and-effect relationship between:

- Hypertension and chronic kidney disease
- Hypertension and heart disease
- Diabetes and chronic kidney disease

It remains the physician's responsibility, however, to document every diagnosis with the highest specificity. Further, if the physician does not want these conditions to be coded as related, the medical record must specifically state they are unrelated.

The physician should clearly document cause-and-effect relationships through the use of linking terms, such as "with," "due to," "secondary to," "associated with," "related to," etc. Best practice is to use descriptors such as "hypertensive" or "diabetic." For example:

- "Diabetic chronic kidney disease, stage 4"
- "Diabetic and hypertensive chronic kidney disease, stage 3"

Documentation and coding examples

Example 1	
Final diagnosis	Renal disease
ICD-10-CM code	N28.9 Disorder of kidney and ureter, unspecified
Comment	A vague and nonspecific diagnostic statement leads to assignment of a vague and nonspecific ICD-10 code.

Example 2	
Final diagnosis	Chronic kidney disease, GFR 40
ICD-10-CM code	N18.9 Chronic kidney disease, unspecified
Comment	GFR is documented, but since the specific stage of CKD is not specified, code N18.9 must be assigned.

Example 3	
Final diagnosis	Stage 5 CKD on hemodialysis
ICD-10-CM code(s)	N18.6 End-stage renal disease Z99.2 Dependence on renal dialysis
Comment	CKD requiring chronic dialysis codes to N18.6 even when not described as end-stage renal disease (ESRD).

ICD-10-CM tips and resources for coders

Coding basics

For accurate and specific diagnosis code assignment, the coder must:

a) Review the entire medical record to verify CKD is a current condition.

b) Note the exact description of CKD documented in the medical record; then, in accordance with ICD-10-CM official coding conventions and guidelines:

c) Search the alphabetic index for that specific description.

d) Verify the code in the tabular list, carefully following all instructional notes.

Coding CKD

CKD classifies to category N18. This category includes instructional notes advising to:

Code first any associated:

diabetic chronic kidney disease (EØ8.22, EØ9.22, E1Ø.22, E11.22, E13.22)

hypertensive chronic kidney disease (I12.-, I13.-)

Use additional code to identify kidney transplant status, if applicable (Z94.Ø).

The ICD-10-CM manual classifies CKD based on the severity of the condition, designated by stages 1-5. The number of each stage corresponds to the fourth character of the ICD-10-CM code as follows:

- CKD stage 1   N18.1
- CKD stage 2   N18.2 (mild)
- CKD stage 3   N18.3 (moderate)
- CKD stage 4   N18.4 (severe)
- CKD stage 5   N18.5 *Excludes1* CKD stage 5 requiring chronic dialysis (N18.6)*
- End-stage renal disease N18.6
  Includes CKD requiring chronic dialysis*
  Use additional code to identify dialysis status (Z99.2)

*These instructional notes indicate CKD requiring chronic dialysis classifies to N18.6 even when the condition is not specifically documented as end-stage renal disease.

Chronic kidney disease, unspecified classifies to code N18.9, which includes:

- Chronic renal disease
- Chronic renal failure not otherwise specified (NOS)
- Chronic renal insufficiency
- Chronic uremia

Coding CKD – continued

If both a stage of CKD and ESRD are documented, assign code N18.6 only.

GFR

GFR is a laboratory blood test used to measure the level of kidney function and determine the stage of kidney disease. It is calculated based on the patient's blood creatinine level, age, body size and gender.

- Note: It is not appropriate to code the stage of CKD based on GFR alone. Rather, the physician must specifically document the stage of CKD.
- If a physician documents the GFR but does not document the stage of CKD (or current chronic hemodialysis), unspecified code N18.9 is assigned.

Renal (kidney) dialysis

Renal dialysis status classifies to code Z99.2, Dependence on renal dialysis. Code Z99.2:

Includes:

- Hemodialysis status
- Peritoneal dialysis status
- Presence of arteriovenous shunt for dialysis
- Renal dialysis status NOS (not otherwise specified)

Excludes1:

- Encounter for fitting and adjustment of dialysis catheter (Z49.Ø-)

Excludes2:

- Noncompliance with renal dialysis (Z91.15)

Chronic kidney disease and associated conditions

According to the ICD-10-CM Official Guidelines for Coding and Reporting (section I.A.15), the word "with" should be interpreted to mean "associated with" or "due to" when it appears in a code title, the alphabetic index or an instructional note in the tabular list. The classification presumes a causal relationship between the two conditions linked by these terms in the alphabetic index or tabular list. These conditions should be coded as related even in the absence of physician documentation explicitly linking them, unless the documentation clearly states the conditions are unrelated. For conditions not specifically linked by these relational terms in the classification, physician documentation must link the conditions to code them as related. The word "with" in the alphabetic index is sequenced immediately following the main term, not in alphabetical order.

CD-10-CM tips and resources for coders

CKD and associated conditions – continued

Based on section I.A.15 of the official guidelines concerning the word "with," the ICD-10-CM classification presumes a cause-and-effect relationship between hypertension and chronic kidney disease, hypertension and heart disease, and diabetes and chronic kidney disease when no other cause is specified.

Hypertensive chronic kidney disease

- Assign codes from category I12, hypertensive chronic kidney disease, when both hypertension and a condition classifiable to category N18, chronic kidney disease, are present.
- In addition to a code from category I12, the appropriate code from category N18 should be used as a secondary code to identify the stage of chronic kidney disease.
- If a patient has hypertensive chronic kidney disease and acute renal failure, an additional code for acute renal failure is required.

Hypertensive heart and chronic kidney disease

- When a medical record supports both hypertensive heart disease and hypertensive kidney disease, assign a code from category I13, hypertensive heart and chronic kidney disease.
  - If heart failure is present, assign an additional code from category I50 to identify the type of heart failure.
  - Assign an additional code from category N18 to identify the stage of chronic kidney disease.
- The codes in category I13, hypertensive heart and chronic kidney disease, are combination codes that include hypertension, heart disease and chronic kidney disease.
  - The *Includes* note at I13 specifies that the conditions included at I11 and I12 are included in I13.
  - If a patient has hypertension, heart disease and chronic kidney disease, use a code from combination category I13 rather than individual codes for hypertension, heart disease and chronic kidney disease or codes from categories I11 or I12.

Diabetes and chronic kidney disease

As noted, diabetes and chronic kidney disease are linked by the term "with" in the alphabetic index. Therefore, these two conditions should be coded as related even in the absence of physician documentation explicitly linking them, unless the documentation clearly states the conditions are unrelated.

When a medical record documents CKD as coexisting with both diabetes and hypertension, CKD should be coded as both diabetic CKD and hypertensive CKD, unless documentation specifies CKD is not caused by hypertension and/or diabetes.

CKD and kidney transplant status

Patients who have undergone kidney transplant still may have some form of CKD because the kidney transplant may not fully restore kidney function. Therefore, the presence of CKD alone does not constitute a transplant complication. When there is no documentation of kidney transplant complication:

- Assign the appropriate code from category N18 for the patient's stage of CKD and code Z94.0, kidney transplant status.

If a transplant complication – such as failure, rejection or other transplant complication – is specifically documented, assign a code from subcategory T86.1-, complications of kidney transplant.

- A code from subcategory T86.1- should not be assigned for post-kidney transplant patients who have CKD unless a transplant complication, such as transplant failure or rejection, is specifically documented.
- If the documentation is unclear as to whether the patient has a complication of the kidney transplant, query the physician for clarification.
- Conditions that affect the function of the transplanted kidney, other than CKD, should be assigned a code from subcategory T86.1- and a secondary code that identifies the complication.

References: American Hospital Association Coding Clinic; ICD-10-CM Official Guidelines for Coding and Reporting; Mayo Clinic; Merck Manual; National Kidney Foundation; WebMD

Clinical overview

Definition

COPD is a broad term that represents a group of chronic, progressive lung diseases that obstruct the airways in the lungs, making it difficult to breathe.

Types

There are two main types of COPD:

- **Emphysema** (slowly progressive destruction of the lung tissue, which loses its elasticity and ability to expand and contract)
- **Chronic bronchitis** (long-term, chronic inflammation and cough with mucus, resulting in narrowing and blockage of the airways)

Note: Most people with COPD have a combination of both conditions.

Causes/risk factors

- Smoking (the No. 1 cause)
- Long-term exposure to environmental irritants (toxic fumes, dust, air pollution, secondhand smoke, etc.)
- History of serious childhood respiratory infections
- Gastroesophageal reflux disease (GERD), which can worsen COPD or may even cause it
- In rare cases, it is thought that genetics – specifically, a deficiency of alpha-1 antitrypsin (AAT), a protein produced in the liver – may play a role

Signs and symptoms

- Chronic cough or cough with large amounts of mucus
- Shortness of breath that is worse with exertion
- Wheezing and chest tightness
- Fatigue

Periodic worsening or "flare-ups" of symptoms are called exacerbations, which can range from mild to life-threatening.

Complications/risks

- Frequent respiratory infections
- Pulmonary hypertension (high blood pressure in the arteries of the lungs)
- Heart problems
- Lung cancer
- Depression
- Weight loss

Diagnostic tools

- Medical history and physical exam
- Pulmonary function tests
- Imaging tests (chest X-ray, CT scan)
- Arterial blood gas analysis
- Pulse oximetry (measures oxygen saturation in the blood)
- Sputum evaluation

Treatment

There is no cure for COPD, and lung damage caused by COPD is not reversible. Treatment is aimed at slowing the progression, managing the symptoms and preventing complications. Treatments include:

- Smoking cessation
- Avoidance of environmental irritants
- Medications
- Pulmonary rehabilitation
- Oxygen therapy
- Influenza and pneumonia immunization
- Regular exercise
- Balanced nutrition
- Surgery (in rare instances): removal of damaged lung tissue or lung transplant

Bronchiectasis is not a type of COPD

COPD and bronchiectasis are two separate chronic lung conditions that can coexist. Although there are some similarities between the two, there also are some important differences and the conditions are treated differently.

- COPD includes a range of chronic, progressive, obstructive lung diseases usually caused by smoking and other environmental factors.
- Bronchiectasis is usually caused by inflammation and infection of the small airways (bronchi), which results in thickening and scarring of walls of the bronchi. This airway damage prevents the natural clearing of mucus; thus, mucus accumulates and creates an environment in which bacteria can grow. This leads to a recurring cycle of inflammation and infection that can cause even more damage to the airways.
  - Over time, the damaged airways lose their ability to effectively move air in and out, resulting in lack of adequate oxygen reaching vital organs. This can lead to serious health problems, such as respiratory failure and heart failure.

Documentation tips for physicians

Abbreviations

A good rule of thumb for any medical record is to limit – or avoid altogether – the use of abbreviations. While COPD is a commonly accepted medical abbreviation for chronic obstructive pulmonary disease, best practice is as follows:

- The initial notation of an abbreviation should be spelled out in full with the abbreviation in parentheses: "Chronic obstructive pulmonary disease (COPD)."
- Subsequent mention of the condition can be made using the abbreviation.

Subjective

In the subjective section of the office note, document the presence or absence of any current symptoms related to chronic obstructive pulmonary disease (e.g., shortness of breath, cough, fatigue, etc.).

Objective

In the objective section of the office note, document any current associated physical exam finding (e.g., decreased breath sounds, wheezing, etc.) and related diagnostic test results.

Suspected versus confirmed

- Do not document a suspected COPD condition as if it were confirmed. Instead, document the signs and symptoms in the absence of a confirmed diagnosis.
- Do not describe a confirmed COPD diagnosis with terms that imply uncertainty (such as "probable," "apparently," "likely" or "consistent with").

Final impression

- It is appropriate to include the COPD diagnosis in the final diagnostic statement, even in the absence of specific treatment of the condition on an individual date of service. American Hospital Association (AHA) Coding Clinic advises COPD is a chronic systemic condition that almost always affects patient care, treatment or management. Therefore, it is appropriate to document the COPD diagnosis in the final assessment as a current, coexisting condition.
- The abbreviation COPD is broad and nonspecific, it does not identify the particular type of COPD or any associated condition. It is important to document the COPD condition with the highest level of specificity.

Final impression – continued

- Examples of COPD described with greater specificity:
  - Acute exacerbation of chronic obstructive bronchitis with asthma
  - Emphysema with chronic bronchitis
  - Chronic obstructive asthma
- Document the current status of the COPD condition (stable, worsening, improved, followed by pulmonologist, etc.).

Treatment plan

- Document a clear and concise treatment plan for COPD, linking related medications to the diagnosis.
- Include orders for diagnostic testing.
- Indicate in the office note to whom or where the referral or consultation is made or from whom consultation advice is requested, if referrals are made or consultations requested.
- Document when the patient will be seen again, even if only on an as-needed basis.

Documentation and coding examples

Example 1	
Final diagnosis	COPD
ICD-10-CM code	J44.9 Chronic obstructive pulmonary disease, unspecified
Comment	A vague and nonspecific condition description leads to assignment of a vague and nonspecific ICD-10 code.

Example 2	
Final diagnosis	Emphysema
ICD-10-CM code	J43.9 Emphysema, unspecified
Comment	Emphysema is a more specific description of COPD.

Example 3	
Final diagnosis	COPD with emphysema
ICD-10-CM code	J43.9 Emphysema, unspecified
Comment	Emphysema is a more specific type of COPD. Following the coding path in the ICD-10-CM manual, emphysema with no mention of chronic bronchitis codes to J43.9.

ICD-10-CM tips and resources for coders

Coding basics

COPD and its associated conditions classify to the following categories:

- J43 Emphysema
- J44 Other chronic obstructive pulmonary disease
- J45 Asthma

Multiple instructional notes appear under each of these categories. To ensure accurate and specific diagnosis code assignment, the coder must note the exact diagnosis description in the medical record; then, in accordance with ICD-10-CM official coding conventions and guidelines:

a) Search the alphabetic index for that specific description; and then

b) Verify the code in the tabular list, following all instructional notes.

COPD

COPD classifies to category J44 with a fourth character required as follows to provide further specificity:

- J44.Ø COPD with acute lower respiratory infection
  Use additional code to identify the infection
- J44.1 COPD with (acute) exacerbation
  Includes *d*ecompensated COPD and
  Decompensated COPD with (acute) exacerbation
  Excludes2 COPD with acute bronchitis (J44.Ø)
- Unspecified COPD codes to J44.9.

COPD with coexisting asthma

Category J44 has an instructional note advising to "code also type of asthma, if applicable (J45.-)".

- Asthma classifies to category J45 with fourth, fifth and sixth characters to specify the particular type of asthma.
- Unspecified asthma codes to J45.9Ø9.
- COPD with asthma codes to J44.9 and J45.9Ø9.
- When a medical record documents both acute exacerbation of asthma and status asthmaticus, only the code for the more severe condition (status asthmaticus) should be assigned.

Emphysema

Emphysema is a more specific description of COPD that classifies to category J43. A fourth character is required to specify the particular type of emphysema. Please note:

- Emphysema documented with coexisting chronic bronchitis classifies to category J44.
- Emphysema without mention of chronic bronchitis classifies to category J43.

COPD with exacerbation and/or acute bronchitis

Exacerbation of COPD is a periodic worsening, flare-up or decompensation of symptoms. An acute exacerbation is not equal to an infection superimposed on COPD (although COPD exacerbation may be triggered by an infection).

- Code J44.1, COPD with exacerbation, has an *Excludes2* note advising code J44.Ø (COPD with acute bronchitis) is not part of the condition represented by code J44.1.
  - This indicates it is acceptable to assign both codes when the medical record shows both conditions currently coexist.
- The record does not have to specifically state the exacerbation is acute to assign code J44.1, as "acute" is enclosed in parentheses as a nonessential modifier – a word that may be present or absent in the statement of a disease without affecting the code to which it is assigned. "Acute" is inherent to exacerbation.

COPD with acute bronchitis (an acute infection) is coded:

- J44.Ø Chronic obstructive pulmonary disease with acute lower respiratory infection
- J2Ø.9 Acute bronchitis, unspecified

COPD with coexisting bronchiectasis

Even though COPD and bronchiectasis are different and separate lung diseases, the ICD-10-CM classification indicates when a record documents COPD co-existing with bronchiectasis, only a code from category J47 is assigned.

In the alphabetic index, bronchiectasis does not appear under **Disease**, pulmonary. However, the coder is advised to see also **Disease**, lung. This leads the coder to **Disease** → lung → obstructive → with → bronchiectasis J47.9.

- Category J47, bronchiectasis, has multiple instructional notes and fourth characters to provide greater specificity.
- Category J44 *Excludes1* COPD with bronchiectasis and directs the coder to category J47.

Other reminders

- Pneumonia is not an acute exacerbation of COPD. When these two conditions coexist, code them separately.
- Hypoxia is not inherent in COPD. When COPD is documented with hypoxia, code RØ9.Ø2, hypoxemia, may be assigned as an additional diagnosis.

References: American Hospital Association Coding Clinic; COPD Foundation; ICD-10-CM Official Guidelines for Coding and Reporting; Mayo Clinic; MedlinePlus; National Heart, Lung and Blood Institute; WebMD

Clinical overview

Definitions

- **Deep vein thrombosis (DVT):** The presence of a blood clot in a deep vein
- **Thrombophlebitis:** Inflammation of a vein caused by or associated with a blood clot
- **Thrombus:** A blood clot that develops inside a blood vessel and stays in place
- **Embolus:** A blood clot that develops inside a blood vessel and subsequently breaks loose and travels to another location
- **Pulmonary embolus (embolism):** A deep vein thrombosis that breaks loose and travels to the lungs

Additional background

A blood clot occurs when blood thickens from a liquid state and hardens into a solid mass.

Most blood clots form in the lower extremities, but they can form in the upper extremities or other locations.

Blood clots can form in superficial veins that are close to the surface, but these are usually not dangerous, as they do not break loose and travel to other locations.

Causes

- Damage to inner lining of a vein (due to injury, inflammation, immune response, etc.)
- Sluggish blood flow (due to prolonged inactivity, such as immobility after surgery or prolonged sitting while traveling)
- Any condition that causes blood to be thicker than normal (e.g., certain medications or medical conditions that increase blood clotting)

Signs and symptoms of current DVT/thrombophlebitis

Often, there are no signs or symptoms. Typically, signs and symptoms develop when there is inflammation associated with the deep vein thrombosis (this is known as thrombophlebitis). These symptoms may include:

- Edema (swelling of affected extremity)
- Pain or tenderness in the affected extremity (positive Homans' sign – pain in the calf or behind the knee with passive flexion of the foot in an upward direction – may indicate the presence of a deep vein thrombosis)
- Increased warmth or redness

Diagnostic tools

- Medical history and physical exam
- Ultrasound/Doppler
- Venography (dye is injected into the vein followed by X-ray of the extremity)
- D-dimer test (measures a substance in the blood that is released when a blood clot dissolves)
- MRI and CT scanning are used less frequently

Main goals of treatment

- Prevent blood clot from enlarging
- Prevent blood clot from breaking loose and traveling to another location
- Prevent future blood clots

Treatment

Medications

- Anticoagulants (blood thinners) decrease the blood's clotting ability and prevent existing clots from getting bigger (blood thinners do not break up existing clots; existing clots usually dissolve with time). Anticoagulant therapy may be used for three to six months or longer, or indefinitely, to prevent recurrence of blood clots. Anticoagulants include:
  - Heparin – acts immediately to thin the blood
  - Coumadin/warfarin – starts to work within three to four days
  - Low-molecular-weight heparins (enoxaparin/Lovenox, dalteparin/Fragmin or tinzaparin/Innohep)
  - Newer advances in drug therapies, such as fondaparinux (Arixtra), rivaroxaban (Xarelto)
- Thrombin inhibitors interfere with the blood-clotting process; they may be used for patients who cannot take heparin.
- Thrombolytics break up blood clots quickly; they are used only in life-threatening situations, as they can cause sudden bleeding.

Compression stockings

Vena cava filter (to catch clots that break loose to prevent them from traveling to the lungs or other locations)

Surgery to remove clot (rarely used)

Documentation tips for physicians

Abbreviations

A good rule of thumb for any medical record is to limit – or avoid altogether – the use of abbreviations. While DVT is a commonly accepted medical abbreviation for deep vein thrombosis, best documentation practice is as follows:

- The initial notation of an abbreviation or acronym should be spelled out in full with the abbreviation/acronym in parentheses — e.g., "deep vein thrombosis (DVT)."
- Subsequent mention of the condition can be made using the abbreviation or acronym.

Subjective

The subjective section of the office note should document the presence of any current symptoms related to deep vein thrombosis (e.g., pain, swelling, redness, etc.).

Objective

The objective section of the office note should include any current associated physical exam findings (e.g., edema, redness, warmth, related diagnostic testing results, etc.).

Current versus "history of"

- A current DVT should not be described anywhere in the record as "history of" DVT. In diagnosis coding, the description "history of" means DVT is historical and no longer exists.
- A deep vein thrombosis that occurred in the past and is no longer present should not be documented in the final assessment as if it is current (assessment: "DVT"). Rather, in this scenario, it is appropriate to describe DVT as "history of" along with specification that the condition is no longer current.

Suspected versus confirmed

- Do not document a suspected deep vein thrombosis as if it were confirmed. Instead, document the signs and symptoms in the absence of a confirmed diagnosis.
- Do not describe a confirmed DVT with terms that imply uncertainty (such as "probable," "apparently," "likely" or "consistent with").

Final assessment/impression

Describe DVT with the highest level of specificity (e.g., acute, chronic, recurrent, historical, exact location, including laterality).

The American Heart Association advises generally a thrombus is referred to as "acute" within the first two weeks after the thrombus forms; "subacute" when more than two weeks and potentially up to six months after thrombus forms; or "chronic" once the thrombus is more than six months old.

- A coder cannot clinically interpret these time frames to determine whether DVT is acute or chronic. Code assignment must strictly correlate with the specific DVT description documented in the medical record.

When a patient is on long-term anticoagulant therapy related to DVT, accurate code assignment requires the physician to clearly link this therapy to the DVT diagnosis and to state the purpose of anticoagulant therapy in the individual case – i.e., whether this therapy is:

a) Part of active treatment of a current acute, current subacute or current chronic DVT, versus
b) Prophylactic treatment related to a historical DVT (to prevent a recurrence).

Best practice is to specifically state whether DVT is acute, chronic or historical and the purpose of associated anticoagulant therapy.

Note: Chronic anticoagulant therapy does not equal a diagnosis of chronic deep vein thrombosis or a coagulation defect.

DVT can occur with or without inflammation.

- Deep vein thrombosis is rarely an acute finding without the associated inflammation that occurs with thrombophlebitis.
- Do not document simply "DVT" when there is also associated thrombophlebitis. Document both conditions to the highest level of specificity. Example: "Acute DVT of the right femoral vein with associated thrombophlebitis."

Plan

Document a specific and concise treatment plan for DVT, including the purpose of any associated long-term anticoagulant therapy and the date of the patient's next appointment.

ICD-10-CM tips and resources for coders

Coding basics

For accurate and specific diagnosis code assignment, the coder must:

a) Review the entire medical record to verify DVT is a current condition and not historical.

b) Note the exact description of the DVT or related condition documented in the medical record; then, in accordance with ICD-10-CM official coding conventions and guidelines:

c) Search the alphabetic index for that specific description.

d) Verify the code in the tabular list, following all instructional notes.

Phlebitis and thrombophlebitis

- Phlebitis and thrombophlebitis of deep vessels of the lower extremities classify to category I8Ø. Fourth, fifth and sixth characters specify the exact location, including the blood vessel affected and laterality.
  - o Review all instructional notes under category I8Ø.
- Category I8Ø excludes (*Excludes1*) venous embolism and thrombosis of lower extremities (I82.4-, I82.5-, I82.81-). An *Excludes1* note indicates that the code excluded should not be used at the same time as the code above the *Excludes1* note.
- When a final diagnosis is stated simply "DVT" but the body of the record documents signs and symptoms that are associated with thrombophlebitis (swelling, erythema, pain and induration), the physician should be queried for clarification and an addendum/ correction created when indicated.

Deep vein thrombosis (DVT)

- Acute embolism and thrombosis of deep veins of the lower extremities classify to subcategory I82.4.
  - o Subcategory I82.4 includes deep vein thrombosis not otherwise specified (NOS) and DVT NOS.
  - o When a medical record supports a current final diagnosis stated simply "deep vein thrombosis" or "DVT" (with no further description or specification), assign code I82.4Ø9, acute embolism and thrombosis of unspecified deep veins of unspecified lower extremity.

Deep vein thrombosis (DVT) – continued

- Chronic embolism and thrombosis of deep veins of the lower extremities classify to subcategory I82.5. For both subcategories, I82.4 and I82.5, fifth and sixth characters are required to specify the exact location – the particular vein affected and laterality (right, left or bilateral).
- There are no specific timelines for when DVT becomes chronic. Code assignment is based solely on the physician's specific description of the condition.
- Acute and chronic embolism and thrombosis of deep veins of the upper extremity classify to subcategories I82.6 (acute) and I82.7 (chronic), with fifth and sixth characters required to specify the site (the particular deep vein affected and laterality).

Long-term anticoagulation therapy

- Z79.Ø1 is assigned for long-term (current) use of anticoagulants.
- Query the physician for clarification when a medical record documents long-term anticoagulant therapy related to DVT but does not specify whether the long-term anticoagulant therapy is being used as:
  a) Active treatment of a current acute, current sub-acute, or current chronic DVT or deep vein thrombophlebitis, versus
  b) Prophylactic treatment of a historical DVT with the goal of preventing recurrence.
- Chronic anticoagulant use (Z79.Ø1) and chronic DVT (subcategory I82.5) are not one and the same.

History of DVT

- Z86.718 represents a personal history of venous thrombosis and embolism.

References: American Heart Association; American Hospital Association Coding Clinic; ICD-10-CM Official Guidelines for Coding and Reporting; Mayo Clinic; MedlinePlus; Merck Manual; National Heart, Lung and Blood Institute

Clinical overview

Definition

Diabetes mellitus is a chronic, lifelong disease that involves impaired metabolism of carbohydrate, protein and fat. It is marked by high levels of sugar in the blood due to insufficient secretion of insulin by the pancreas, tissue resistance to insulin produced by the pancreas or both.

Background

Normally, sugar from food is converted to glucose, which enters the bloodstream and is used by the body for energy. Insulin produced in the pancreas "unlocks" the tissue cells in the body, allowing glucose to enter to provide fuel and energy for the cells.

Types

- **Type 1 diabetes mellitus** – Usually (but not always) diagnosed in childhood. The pancreas produces little to no insulin and daily insulin injections are required. The exact cause of Type 1 diabetes mellitus is not known.
- **Latent autoimmune diabetes in adults (LADA)** – Sometimes referred to as diabetes mellitus Type 1.5. LADA is a more slowly progressive variation of Type 1 diabetes and is often misdiagnosed as Type 2 because it occurs at a later age. Unlike Type 2 diabetes mellitus, LADA does not have insulin resistance. LADA is characterized by age, a lack of family history of Type 2 diabetes, a gradual increase in insulin requirements, positive antibodies and decreasing ability to produce insulin.
- **Type 2 diabetes mellitus** – Far more common than Type 1, this usually occurs in adulthood. The pancreas does not produce enough insulin to maintain normal glucose levels, often because the body tissues do not respond well to insulin (insulin resistance). In some cases, daily insulin injections are required. The exact cause of Type 2 diabetes mellitus is not known, but excess weight and inactivity appear to be contributing factors.
- **Secondary diabetes mellitus** – Always caused by another condition, such as malignant neoplasm of the pancreas, pancreatectomy, adverse drug effects or poisoning.

Risk factors for Type 2 diabetes mellitus

- Age (older than 45 years)
- Obesity
- High cholesterol levels
- Polycystic ovary syndrome in women
- History of gestational diabetes or delivering a baby weighing more than 9 pounds
- Physical inactivity
- Heart disease
- Family history of diabetes
- History of glucose intolerance
- Ethnicity (certain ethnic groups are at higher risk)

Signs and symptoms

- Frequent urination (polyuria)
- Excessive thirst (polydipsia)
- Excessive hunger (polyphagia)
- Unusual weight loss
- Fatigue
- Irritability
- Blurry vision

Complications

Acute complications

- Infections
- Stroke
- Diabetic ketoacidosis – an acute life-threatening condition requiring immediate medical attention. Develops when cells in the body are unable to get the sugar (glucose) they need for energy. The body begins to break down fat and muscle for energy; this process produces ketones, which enter the bloodstream and cause a chemical imbalance. Severe diabetic ketoacidosis carries a coma risk and even death.

Long-term complications (tend to be chronic, but can be reversible in some cases)
- Diabetic neuropathy
- Diabetic retinopathy
- Hypertension
- Atherosclerotic peripheral vascular disease
- Diabetic nephropathy
- Hyperlipidemia
- Coronary artery disease

Diagnostic tools

- Medical history and physical exam
- Urinalysis
- Blood tests (fasting or random blood sugar, glucose tolerance tests, glycohemoglobin, metabolic profiles)

Treatment

- Treatment depends on the type of diabetes. May include insulin injections or oral medications. Other treatments: dietary management; regular exercise; weight control, blood pressure and cholesterol; close monitoring of blood glucose levels; diabetes education; and monitoring for complication.

Documentation tips for physicians

Abbreviations

Limit or avoid acronyms and abbreviations. DM is a commonly accepted medical abbreviation for diabetes mellitus but can represent other medical conditions (diastolic murmur or distal metastasis). The meaning of an abbreviation can often be determined based on context, but not always. Best practice is to spell out the diagnosis in full in the final assessment/impression.

Subjective

In the subjective section of the office note, document the presence or absence of all current symptoms related to DM. If there are no current symptoms, this section should show the patient was screened for symptoms.

Objective

In the objective section, document current exam findings related to DM or its manifestations. If none, clearly show the patient was evaluated for related findings.

Final assessment/impression

Document DM with the highest level of specificity. Include all of the following:

- **Type or cause:**
  - Type 1, Type 2, due to drugs or chemicals (specify causative drug or chemical), due to other disease or condition (specify causative disease or condition), other specified type (specify type)
- **All complications or manifestations** with clear cause-and-effect linkage*
- **Current status of diabetes control** – if uncontrolled, specify hyperglycemia versus hypoglycemia
- **"Long-term current use of insulin"** – cannot be coded from a medication list alone; diagnosis should be documented in the final assessment/ impression with all of the following information:
  - Name of the insulin being used
  - Clear linkage of insulin therapy to diabetes
  - The dosage regimen that shows regular and routine insulin use with ongoing refills

  Example: "Continue Levemir FlexTouch 14 units every day at bedtime for diabetes mellitus, 3 refills"

Plan

- Document a specific and concise treatment plan.
- Include the date of the patient's next visit.

Major ICD-10-CM alerts and reminders

- Avoid vague descriptions of the current status of diabetes control, such as "inadequately controlled," "out of control" or "poorly controlled" (which all default to coding as hyperglycemia). Remember that ICD-10-CM requires the physician to specify "uncontrolled" as either hyperglycemia or hypoglycemia.
- ICD-10-CM presumes cause-and-effect linkage between diabetes and certain conditions unless the physician specifically indicates the conditions are not related. Conditions that appear in the alphabetic index as indented subterms under the various types of "diabetes, with" are coded as diabetic complications, even in the absence of physician documentation explicitly linking them, unless the documentation clearly indicates these conditions are not caused by diabetes — for example, by stating:
  - Actual nondiabetes-related cause
  - Cause is not diabetes
  - Diabetes is without complications
  - Cause is unknown

  Excerpt from alphabetic index:
  Diabetes, diabetic (mellitus) (sugar) E11.9
    with
      amyotrophy E11.44
      arthropathy NEC E11.618
      autonomic (poly)neuropathy E11.43
      cataract E11.36
      Charcot joints E11.610
      chronic kidney disease E11.22

(This example list is not all-inclusive. For complete lists, see alphabetic index under the various types of diabetes followed by indented subterm "with.")

It remains the physician's responsibility to document every diagnosis with the highest specificity.

*Best documentation practice: Describe each complication with the descriptor "diabetic," even when there are multiple complications. Example: "Diabetes mellitus Type 2, uncontrolled due to hyperglycemia, with diabetic peripheral neuropathy and diabetic foot ulcer."

Electronic medical records (EMR) reminders

- A diagnosis of "diabetes mellitus with other manifestation" is incomplete unless the record clearly specifies the "other" manifestation.
- Avoid conflicting or contradictory information. Examples: The EMR documents Type 1 *and* Type 2, controlled *and* uncontrolled, with *and* without complications.

ICD-10-CM tips and resources for coders

Coding basics

For accurate and specific diagnosis code assignment, the coder must review the entire medical record and note the exact description of diabetes and all related conditions documented in the medical record. Then, in accordance with the ICD-10-CM official coding conventions and guidelines:

a) Search the alphabetic index for that specific description.

b) Verify the code in the tabular list, carefully following all instructional notes.

Coding diabetes mellitus

In ICD-10-CM, the codes for diabetes mellitus begin with the letter E and are found in Chapter 4: Endocrine, Nutritional, and Metabolic Diseases. The diabetes codes are combination codes that identify:

a) The type of diabetes mellitus

b) The body system affected

c) The particular complications that affect each body system

Diabetes mellitus is coded from categories E08 – E13:

E08	Diabetes mellitus due to underlying cause
E09	Drug or chemical induced diabetes mellitus
E10	Type 1 diabetes mellitus
E11	Type 2 diabetes mellitus
E13	Other specified diabetes mellitus

Fourth, fifth and, in some cases, sixth characters are required to further describe the diabetic condition with the highest level of specificity.

- "Code first" and "use additional code" notes are present for some of the diabetes mellitus categories and subcategories.
    - The underlying condition is sequenced first, followed by the complication/manifestation.
    - The "use additional code" note appears at the etiology code and the "code first" note at the complication/manifestation code.

- The *"Excludes1"* note (meaning "not coded here") appears under all the diabetes mellitus categories. An *Excludes1* note indicates that the code excluded should never be used at the same time as the code above the *Excludes1* note.

Type of diabetes mellitus

- When the type of diabetes mellitus is not documented in the medical record, the default is Type 2, which classifies to category E11.

- Diabetes mellitus Type 1.5 with no further specification should be coded to category E10, Type 1 diabetes, which includes diabetes due to an autoimmune process.

Current status of diabetes control

- There is no ICD-10-CM code for diabetes mellitus described as "uncontrolled" without specification of hypoglycemia versus hyperglycemia. If physician query is not possible, the best available option is to code to diabetes, by type, with fourth character -.8.

- Per the alphabetic index, diabetes mellitus described as "inadequately controlled," "out of control" or "poorly controlled" defaults to diabetes, by type, with hyperglycemia.

Diabetic complications/manifestations

Diabetic patients often experience one or more complications of diabetes that particularly affect the eyes, the feet, the kidneys, the nervous system and the circulatory system. These complications can occur at any time in the course of diabetes.

- A patient may have multiple diabetic complications in more than one body area or system. To fully describe all of the diabetes complications that are present, assign as many codes as needed from categories E08 – E13 and within each particular subcategory. Codes are sequenced based on the reason for the encounter.

- As noted in the documentation section on page 2 of this guideline, ICD-10-CM presumes cause-and-effect linkage between diabetes and certain conditions that appear in the alphabetic index as indented subterms under the various types of "diabetes, with." These conditions are coded as diabetic complications, even in the absence of documentation explicitly linking them, unless the documentation clearly indicates these conditions are not caused by diabetes — for example, by stating:
    - The actual nondiabetes-related cause
    - That the cause is not diabetes
    - That diabetes is without complications
    - That the cause is unknown

ICD-10-CM tips and resources for coders

Example from alphabetic index:

Diabetes, diabetic (mellitus) (sugar) E11.9

  with

    amyotrophy E11.44

    arthropathy NEC E11.618

    autonomic (poly)neuropathy E11.43

    cataract E11.36

    Charcot joints E11.61Ø

    chronic kidney disease E11.22

(This example list is not all-inclusive. For complete lists, see alphabetic index under the various types of diabetes followed by indented subterm "with.")

For conditions not specifically linked by the word "with" in the code title, alphabetic index or tabular list, the documentation must clearly link the conditions to code them as related.

Diabetes mellitus (DM), hypertension (HTN) and chronic kidney disease (CKD)

Medical record documents current diagnoses of CKD, HTN and DM but does not document cause-and-effect linkage between any combination of the three:

- Presume CKD is linked to both conditions and code both hypertensive CKD and diabetic CKD.

Medical record documents DM coexisting with hypertensive CKD with no cause-and-effect linkage between DM and CKD:

- Code only hypertensive CKD; do not code diabetic CKD. The descriptor "hypertensive" specifically identifies hypertension as the cause of CKD. CKD should not be coded as diabetic since the physician has specifically documented a different cause (HTN).

Medical record documents HTN coexisting with diabetic CKD with no cause-and-effect linkage between HTN and CKD:

- Code only diabetic CKD; do not code hypertensive CKD. The descriptor "diabetic" specifically identifies diabetes as the cause of CKD. CKD should not be coded as hypertensive since the physician has specifically documented a different cause (DM).

Insulin use and oral hypoglycemic drugs

- Long-term (current) use of insulin does not affect the selection of the type of diabetes – insulin use does not automatically mean the patient is Type 1. (Some Type 2 diabetics use insulin.)

Insulin use and oral hypoglycemic drugs – continued

- If the documentation in a medical record does not indicate the type of diabetes but does indicate the patient uses insulin, assign category E11, Type 2 diabetes mellitus.
- Assign code Z79.4, long-term (current) use of insulin, or Z79.84, long-term (current) use of oral hypoglycemic drugs, to indicate the patient uses insulin or hypoglycemic drugs. Code Z79.4 should not be assigned if insulin is given temporarily to bring a Type 2 patient's blood sugar under control during an encounter.
- Code Z79.4 should not be coded from a medication list. Assign code Z79.4 when the final assessment or impression clearly documents long-term, current use of insulin that is clearly linked to diabetes, along with the dosage regimen that shows regular and routine insulin use with ongoing prescription refills.
- When the record supports long-term, current use of both oral hypoglycemic medications and insulin, only code Z79.4 for long-term, current use of insulin should be assigned.

Secondary diabetes mellitus

Secondary diabetes mellitus is always caused by another condition or event (e.g., cystic fibrosis, malignant neoplasm of pancreas, pancreatectomy, adverse effect of drug or poisoning). Secondary diabetes and associated complications/manifestations classify to the following categories:

EØ8	Diabetes mellitus due to underlying condition
EØ9	Drug or chemical induced diabetes mellitus
E13	Other specified diabetes mellitus (identify)

- Sequencing of the secondary diabetes codes in relationship to codes for the cause of the diabetes is based on the tabular list instructions for categories EØ8, EØ9 and E13.

- Secondary diabetes mellitus due to pancreatectomy (lack of insulin due to surgical removal of all or part of the pancreas) codes to E89.1, postprocedural hypoinsulinemia. Assign a code from category E13 and a code from subcategory Z9Ø.41-, acquired absence of pancreas, as additional codes.

ICD-10-CM tips and resources for coders

Secondary diabetes mellitus – continued

- Secondary diabetes mellitus due to drugs may be caused by an adverse effect of correctly administered medications, poisoning or sequela of poisoning. See ICD-10-CM Official Guidelines for Coding and Reporting:
  - Section I.C.19.e for coding adverse effects and poisoning
  - Section I.C.20 for external cause code reporting

Prediabetes and borderline diabetes

Prediabetes and borderline diabetes mellitus both classify to code R73.Ø3, prediabetes.

Diabetes mellitus resolved

Generally speaking, diabetes mellitus is a chronic, lifelong condition. However, diabetes mellitus may be described as resolved in some cases. For example:

- Type 1 diabetes mellitus resolved following pancreas transplant
- Type 2 diabetes mellitus resolved after significant weight loss following gastric bypass surgery

When a medical record documents diabetes mellitus as resolved, the condition cannot be coded as current.

References: American Heart Association; Dorland's Medical Dictionary; MedlinePlus; ICD-10-CM Official Guidelines for Coding and Reporting; Mayo Clinic

Heart Failure

Clinical overview

Definition

Heart failure is a condition in which the heart muscle is unable to pump enough blood through the heart to meet the body's needs for blood and oxygen.

Background

The heart has four chambers: the upper chambers (right and left atria) and the lower chambers (right and left ventricles). Oxygen-rich blood travels from the lungs to the heart, where it is pumped out to the rest of the body. Oxygen-poor blood returns from the body to the heart and back to the lungs to again receive oxygen. When the heart functions properly, all four chambers beat and pump blood effectively in an organized way. When heart failure develops, the heart is no longer able to pump blood effectively. In the early stages, the heart is able to compensate in these ways:

- The heart chambers enlarge, and the heart develops more muscle mass.
- The heart pumps faster and diverts blood away from less important areas of the body to the heart and brain.
- Blood vessels narrow to keep blood pressure up.

Eventually, the heart no longer can compensate, and signs and symptoms of heart failure develop.

Types

- **Left-sided heart failure**: The most common form of heart failure, it involves a decreased ability of the left ventricle to effectively pump blood out to the rest of the body. Fluid may back up in the lungs, causing shortness of breath.
- **Right-sided heart failure**: The right side no longer pumps effectively, and blood backs up in the body's veins, causing swelling in the tissues. This form is usually due to left-sided heart failure.
- **Systolic failure**: The left ventricle loses its ability to contract normally, thus it cannot effectively pump blood out of the heart to the body.
- **Diastolic failure**: The left ventricle loses its ability to relax normally; thus, it cannot fill with blood during the resting period between beats.
- **Congestive heart failure (CHF)**: A slowing of blood flow out of the heart that occurs with heart failure also can cause blood returning to the heart to slow and back up, resulting in congestion in body tissues. This leads to edema – swelling – in the lower extremities and congestion in the lungs that interferes with breathing.

Causes/risk factors

- Smoking
- Hypertension
- Lung disease
- Past heart attack
- Coronary artery disease
- Abnormal heart valves
- Obesity
- Diabetes
- Congenital heart disease
- Diseases of heart muscle
- Heart arrhythmias
- Other medical conditions

Signs and symptoms

- Edema/swelling of feet, ankles, abdomen
- Increased heart rate or palpitations
- Shortness of breath
- Fatigue
- Confusion
- Decreased urine
- Difficulty sleeping
- Decreased exercise tolerance
- Persistent cough or wheezing
- Weight gain
- Loss of appetite
- Indigestion
- Nausea and vomiting

Diagnostic tools

- Medical history and physical exam
- Lab testing, including B-type natriuretic peptide (BNP) lab test: BNP is a substance secreted by the ventricles in response to pressure changes in the heart that occur with heart failure. The blood BNP level increases when heart failure gets worse and decreases when heart failure is stable.
- Chest X-ray and electrocardiogram (ECG or EKG)
- Echocardiogram
- Cardiac stress testing and catheterization
- CT or MRI scans
- Nuclear heart scans

Treatment

- Regular monitoring
- Limited salt intake
- Smoking cessation
- Exercise
- Weight control and balanced nutrition
- Treatment of underlying conditions
- Medications (diuretics, beta blockers, angiotensin-converting enzyme inhibitors, digitalis glycosides, angiotensin receptor blockers)
- Pacemaker or implantable cardioverter defibrillator
- Heart pumps (left ventricular assist devices)
- Heart transplant

Documentation tips for physicians

Abbreviations

- A good rule of thumb for any medical record is to limit – or avoid altogether – the use of acronyms and abbreviations. "CHF" is a commonly accepted medical abbreviation for congestive heart failure. "HF" is sometimes used to represent heart failure; however, this abbreviation has other meanings. The meaning of an abbreviation often can be determined based on context, but this is not always true. Best practice is to always spell out each diagnosis in full in the final assessment or impression.

Subjective

- The subjective section of the office note should show the patient was asked about symptoms. Document the presence or absence of any current symptoms of heart failure.

Objective

- The objective section of the office note should include any current associated physical exam finding (such as edema, weight gain, shortness of breath, etc.) and results of any related diagnostic testing.

Current versus "history of"

- Do not use the descriptor "history of" to describe current heart failure. In diagnosis coding, the descriptor "history of" implies the condition occurred in the past and is no longer current.
- Temporary or transient heart failure that occurred in the past and is no longer present should not be documented as if it is current.

Final assessment/impression

- Do not document suspected heart failure as if it is confirmed. Rather, document the signs and symptoms in the absence of a confirmed diagnosis.
- For a confirmed current diagnosis of heart failure, do not use descriptors that imply uncertainty (such as "probable," "apparently," "likely" or "consistent with").
- Document heart failure to the highest level of specificity, using all applicable descriptors (congestive, hypertensive, post-operative, acute, chronic, acute-on-chronic, diastolic, systolic, etc.).

Final assessment/impression – continued

- State the cause of heart failure, if known, using terms that clearly show cause and effect (such as "associated with," "due to," "secondary to," "hypertensive," etc.).
- Document the current status of heart failure (stable, worsening, improved, in remission, compensated, etc.).

Plan

- Document a specific and concise treatment plan for heart failure, including date of next appointment.
  - If referrals are made or consultations requested, the office note should indicate to whom or where the referral or consultation is made or from whom consultation advice is requested.

Documentation and coding examples

Example 1	
Final diagnosis	CHF with diastolic dysfunction
ICD-10-CM code	I50.30

Example 2	
Final diagnosis	Acute combined systolic and diastolic congestive heart failure
ICD-10-CM code	I50.41

Example 3	
Final diagnosis	Chronic diastolic CHF, due to hypertension
ICD-10-CM codes	I11.0, I50.32

Example 4	
Final diagnosis	Diastolic dysfunction
ICD-10-CM code	I51.89

Example 5	
Final diagnosis	Hypertensive heart failure
ICD-10-CM codes	I11.0, I50.9

Example 6	
Final diagnosis	Acute on chronic systolic heart failure
ICD-10-CM code	I50.23

Example 7	
Final diagnosis	Exacerbation of CHF, diastolic
ICD-10-CM code	I50.33

ICD-10-CM tips and resources for coders

Basics of coding heart failure

For accurate and specific diagnosis code assignment, the coder must:

a) Review the entire medical record to verify the heart failure condition is current.

b) Note the exact cardiomyopathy description documented in the medical record; then, in accordance with ICD-10-CM official coding conventions and guidelines:

c) Search the alphabetic index for that specific description.

d) Verify the code in the tabular list, following all instructional notes.

Heart failure classifies to category I5Ø. See tabular list for conditions that should be coded first.

- Fourth characters are assigned to specify the type of heart failure.
  - I5Ø.1 Left ventricular failure
  - I5Ø.2 Systolic (congestive) heart failure
  - I5Ø.3 Diastolic (congestive) heart failure
  - I5Ø.4 Combined systolic (congestive) and diastolic (congestive) heart failure
  - I5Ø.9 Heart failure, unspecified
    Excludes2 fluid overload (E87.7Ø)
    Includes
    Biventricular (heart) failure not otherwise specified (NOS)
    Cardiac, heart or myocardial failure NOS
    Congestive heart disease
    Congestive heart failure NOS
    Right ventricular failure (secondary to left heart failure)
- Fifth characters are added to specify acute, chronic or acute-on-chronic combined.

Subcategories I5Ø.2 — I5Ø.4 include the descriptor "congestive" as a nonessential modifier (a supplementary word that may be absent or present in the diagnostic statement without affecting the code number to which it is assigned).

- Therefore, when the final diagnosis lists congestive heart failure along with either systolic or diastolic heart failure, only the code for the type of heart failure is assigned (systolic and/or diastolic).

The terms "heart failure" and "congestive heart failure" often are used interchangeably, even though congestion (pulmonary or systemic fluid buildup) is one feature of heart failure that does not occur in all patients with heart failure. This means that from a clinical standpoint, "heart failure" and "congestive heart failure" are not one and the same.

- Despite this clinical information, in ICD-10-CM, "heart failure" and "congestive heart failure" classify to the same code: I5Ø.9, heart failure, unspecified. Code I5Ø.9 includes congestive heart failure; there is no separate code for CHF.

It is not appropriate to code heart failure based on the coder's own clinical interpretation of documented signs, symptoms or lab values. Rather, code assignment is strictly based on the specific description of heart failure documented by the physician.

Hypertension with heart disease

ICD-10-CM presumes a cause-and-effect relationship between hypertension (HTN) and heart disease and advises these two conditions should be coded as related even in the absence of physician documentation explicitly linking them, unless the documentation specifically indicates they are not related.

HTN with heart conditions classified to I5Ø.- or I51.4–I51.9 are assigned to a code from category I11, hypertensive heart disease.

- Use an additional code from category I5Ø, heart failure, to identify the type of heart failure in those patients with heart failure.
- The same heart conditions (I5Ø.-, I51.4–I51.9) with hypertension are coded separately if the physician has specifically documented a different cause. Sequence according to the circumstances of the admission/encounter.

Hypertensive heart and chronic kidney disease

Assign codes from combination category I13, hypertensive heart and chronic kidney disease, when there is hypertension with both heart and kidney involvement. If heart failure is present, assign an additional code from category I5Ø to identify the type of heart failure. The appropriate code from category N18, chronic kidney disease, should be used as a secondary code with a code from category I13 to identify the stage of chronic kidney disease.

ICD-10-CM tips and resources for coders

Hypertensive heart and chronic kidney disease – continued

The codes in category I13, hypertensive heart and chronic kidney disease, are combination codes that include hypertension, heart disease and chronic kidney disease. The *Includes* note at I13 specifies that the conditions included at I11 and I12 are included together in I13. If a patient has hypertension, heart disease and chronic kidney disease, then a code from I13 should be used, not individual codes for hypertension, heart disease and chronic kidney disease, or codes from I11 or I12.

Heart dysfunction

Heart dysfunction without mention of heart failure codes to I51.89, other ill-defined heart diseases. The coder cannot assume a patient is in heart failure when only "diastolic dysfunction" or "systolic dysfunction" is documented.

Right- and left-sided heart failure

Right-sided heart failure (I5Ø.9) ordinarily follows left-sided failure (I5Ø.1). Code I5Ø.9 includes any left-sided failure that is present; therefore, codes I5Ø.1 and I5Ø.9 are not assigned together for the same episode of care, and code I5Ø.9 takes precedence.

Compensated, decompensated, exacerbation

- "Compensated" heart failure means the heart has developed compensatory mechanisms that permit near-normal heart function.
- "Decompensated" or "exacerbation" both indicate a flare-up (acute phase) of heart failure – an increase in the severity of heart failure or any of its symptoms. When heart failure is described as currently decompensated or exacerbated, it should be coded as acute-on-chronic.

References: American Heart Association; American Hospital Association Coding Clinic; Cleveland Clinic; ICD-10-CM Official Guidelines for Coding and Reporting; Mayo Clinic; MedlinePlus

Clinical overview

Definition

The Diagnostic and Statistical Manual of Mental Disorders, Fifth Edition – Text Revision (DSM-5) of the American Psychiatric Association (APA) advises that major depression is a mental disorder, marked by a depressed mood and loss of interest or pleasure in all activities that lasts for at least two weeks and represents a change from previous functioning.

Causes

The exact cause is not known. Factors that may play a role include:

- Biological differences/physical changes in the brain
- Brain chemicals (called neurotransmitters) that are linked to mood
- Changes in hormone balance
- Genetics/inherited traits
- Life events
- Trauma during early childhood

Signs and symptoms

The DSM-5 provides detailed and specific criteria that must be met to diagnose major depression or major depressive disorder. The specific criteria include the following excerpt:

A. Five (or more) of the following symptoms have been present during the same two-week period and represent a change from previous functioning; at least one of the symptoms is either (1) depressed mood or (2) loss of interest or pleasure.
   Note: Do not include symptoms that are clearly attributable to another medical condition.
   1. Depressed mood most of the day
   2. Markedly diminished interest or pleasure in all, or almost all, activities most of the day
   3. Significant weight loss when not dieting, or weight gain, or decrease or increase in appetite
   4. Insomnia or hypersomnia nearly every day
   5. Psychomotor agitation or retardation
   6. Fatigue or loss of energy
   7. Feelings of worthlessness or excessive or inappropriate guilt (which may be delusional)
   8. Diminished ability to think or concentrate, or indecisiveness
   9. Recurrent thoughts of death (not just fear of dying), recurrent suicidal ideation without a specific plan or a suicide attempt or a specific plan for committing suicide
B. The symptoms cause clinically significant distress or impairment in social, occupational, or other important areas of functioning.
C. The episode is not attributable to the physiological effects of a substance or to another medical condition.

   Criteria A-C represent a major depressive episode.

- **See the DSM-5 for complete information.**

Complications

Major depression that is left untreated can cause complications, such as:

- Alcohol or substance abuse
- Anxiety
- Heart disease or other medical conditions
- Work or school issues
- Family conflicts
- Relationship difficulties
- Social isolation
- Suicide

Diagnostic tools

- Medical history and physical exam
- Laboratory tests to check for and monitor underlying medical conditions
- Psychological evaluation

Treatment

- Medications
- Psychotherapy/mental health counseling
- Electroconvulsive therapy
- Vagus nerve stimulation
- Transcranial magnetic stimulation

Self-help strategies

- Adherence to treatment plan
- Education about depression
- Observation for warning signs
- Exercise and adequate sleep
- Avoidance of alcohol and illicit drugs

Documentation tips for physicians

Abbreviations

- Limit – or avoid altogether – the use of acronyms and abbreviations. While MDD is a commonly accepted medical abbreviation for major depressive disorder, this abbreviation also can be used to represent manic depressive disorder, which classifies to a different diagnosis code. The meaning of an abbreviation can often be determined based on context, but this is not always true. Best practice is to document major depression or major depressive disorder by spelling out the diagnosis in full.

Subjective

- In the subjective section of the office note, document the presence or absence of any current symptoms related to major depressive disorder.

Objective

- The objective section should include any current associated physical exam findings (such as "flat affect," weight loss or gain, etc.).
- If there are no current related exam findings, the objective section should show the patient was evaluated for related findings.

Final assessment/impression

- Document the diagnosis by spelling it out in full.
- Do not use the descriptor "history of" to describe current major depression that is still present, active and ongoing. In diagnosis coding, the phrase "history of" means the condition is historical and no longer exists as a current problem.
- Do not document major depression as if it is current when the condition is truly historical and no longer exists as a current problem.
- Major depression that is in remission but still has impact on patient care, treatment and management should be included in the final assessment or impression with the current status noted as "in remission."
- For a confirmed diagnosis of major depressive disorder or major depression, do not use descriptors that imply uncertainty (such as "probable," "apparently," "likely" or "consistent with").

Final assessment/impression – continued

- Do not document suspected major depressive disorder or major depression as if the diagnosis were confirmed. Document the signs and symptoms in the absence of a confirmed diagnosis.
- Note: ICD-10-CM classifies "depression" without further description as major depression. Therefore, it is critical that physicians document depression as specifically as possible to ensure accurate diagnosis code assignment. Not doing so could result in many patients being erroneously classified as having a major depressive disorder when that is not the case.
- On the other hand, when a diagnosis of major depression is appropriate, not documenting all applicable descriptors will result in inaccurate code assignment. Be sure to include all of the following:
  - Episode – single or recurrent
  - Severity – mild, moderate, severe
  - Presence or absence of psychosis/psychotic features
  - Remission status – partial or full

- **To become familiar with all the descriptors, review the ICD-10-CM manual and the section on page 3 titled "ICD-10-CM tips and resources for coders."**

Plan

- Document a specific and concise treatment plan for major depression, including date of next appointment.
- Document to whom or where referrals are made or from whom consultation advice is requested.

ICD-10-CM tips and resources for coders

Coding major depression

Major depression classifies to the following categories with fourth and fifth characters to provide further specificity (mild, moderate, severe; with or without psychotic features; partial or full remission):

F32 Major depressive disorder, single episode

F32.Ø   Major depressive disorder, single episode, mild

F32.1   Major depressive disorder, single episode, moderate

F32.2   Major depressive disorder, single episode, severe without psychotic features

F32.3   Major depressive disorder, single episode, severe with psychotic features

F32.4   Major depressive disorder, single episode, in partial remission

F32.5   Major depressive disorder, single episode, in full remission

F32.9   Major depressive disorder, single episode, unspecified; includes: depression not otherwise specified (NOS), depressive disorder NOS, major depression NOS

F33 Major depressive disorder, recurrent

F33.Ø   Major depressive disorder, recurrent, mild

F33.1   Major depressive disorder, recurrent, moderate

F33.2   Major depressive disorder, recurrent, severe without psychotic features

F33.3   Major depressive disorder, recurrent, severe with psychotic symptoms

F33.4- Major depressive disorder, recurrent, in remission

    F33.4Ø   Major depressive disorder, recurrent, in remission, unspecified

    F33.41   Major depressive disorder, recurrent, in partial remission

    F33.42   Major depressive disorder, recurrent, in full remission

F33.8   Other recurrent depressive disorders

F33.9   Major depressive disorder, recurrent, unspecified

Other coding tips

- ICD-10-CM code assignment is based on the exact diagnosis as described by the physician in the medical record. Coders are not allowed to make any assumptions based on documented signs and symptoms or other patient work-up that may show that the DSM-5 criteria for major depression are met. Only the physician can assign a diagnosis of major depression based on his or her evaluation of the patient and application of the specific criteria outlined in the DSM-5.

- The abbreviation MDD can have more than one meaning (manic-depressive disorder versus major depressive disorder, which classify to two different ICD-10-CM codes). The diagnosis must be clearly spelled out in full within the record to substantiate the meaning of the abbreviation.

- Situational depression codes to F43.21, adjustment disorder with depressed mood.

References: Diagnostic and Statistical Manual of Mental Disorders, Fifth Edition – Text Revision (DSM-5); Mayo Clinic; ICD-10-CM Official Guidelines for Coding and Reporting; 2008 Risk Adjustment Data Technical Assistance for Medicare Advantage Organizations Participant Guide – Diagnosis Codes and Risk Adjustment

Clinical overview

Definition

A myocardial infarction is a condition in which an artery that supplies blood to the heart is blocked, cutting off the supply of oxygen and nutrients to that area of the heart. As a result, the affected heart tissue dies or is permanently damaged.

Causes

- Atherosclerosis of the coronary arteries, where fatty plaques that build up inside the coronary arteries block blood flow or cause blood clots
- Blood clots
- Sudden severe stress
- Spasms of the coronary arteries

Risk factors

- Age (older than 65)
- Gender (male)
- Diabetes mellitus
- Genetic or hereditary factors
- High blood pressure/hypertension
- Smoking
- High-fat diet
- High cholesterol and triglycerides
- Lack of exercise
- Obesity
- Illicit drug use

Signs and symptoms

There may be no signs or symptoms ("silent" myocardial infarction). When they do occur, the most common signs and symptoms include:

- Chest pain (heaviness, pressure, feeling of a tight band around chest, etc.); pain may radiate to jaw, neck, arm or back
- Indigestion
- Abdominal pain
- Anxiety or feeling of impending doom
- Nausea and vomiting
- Shortness of breath
- Rapid or irregular heartbeat
- Fatigue or lightheadedness
- Sweating

Complications

- Arrhythmias (irregular or abnormal heart rhythms)
- Heart failure
- Cardiomyopathy
- Heart rupture
- Heart valve problems
- Blood clot to lungs (pulmonary embolism) or brain (stroke)

Diagnostic tools

- Medical history and physical exam
- Chest X-ray
- Blood tests
- Electrocardiogram (ECG or EKG)
- Echocardiogram
- Coronary angiography (cardiac catheterization)
- Exercise stress tests
- CT scans and MRI
- Nuclear scans

Treatment

- Medications (anticoagulants or thrombolytics, pain relievers, nitroglycerin, beta blockers, angiotensin-converting enzyme inhibitors, cholesterol-reducing agents)
- Oxygen therapy
- Surgical intervention (coronary angioplasty and stenting, coronary artery bypass grafting)

Myocardial Infarction   ICD-10-CM

Documentation tips for physicians

Abbreviations

- Limit – or avoid altogether – the use of acronyms and abbreviations. While "MI" is a commonly accepted medical abbreviation for myocardial infarction, this abbreviation has other meanings related to cardiac conditions (for example, mitral insufficiency and mitral incompetence). The meaning of an abbreviation often can be determined based on context, but this is not always true. Best practice is to always document myocardial infarction by spelling it out in full.

Site/location

- Specify the site or location within the heart of myocardial infarction, such as anterolateral wall, inferoposterior wall, lateral wall, subendocardial, etc. Also specify the particular coronary artery or arteries involved.

Dates/timelines

Clearly document specific timelines or dates associated with myocardial infarction, as this influences ICD-10-CM code assignment.

- A myocardial infarction that occurred four weeks ago or less is coded as an acute myocardial infarction (still in the acute phase of medical care).
- Encounters after the four-week time frame but with the patient still receiving care related to the myocardial infarction are coded as "aftercare" rather than acute myocardial infarction.
- A myocardial infarction that occurred more than four weeks ago with no current symptoms directly associated with that myocardial infarction and requiring no current care is coded as an "old" or historical myocardial infarction.
- Avoid use of vague descriptions (such as "recent" myocardial infarction), as these descriptions do not specify whether the myocardial infarction occurred less than or more than four weeks ago. If describing myocardial infarction as "recent," include the specific date or timeline, as in "recent myocardial infarction on June 1, 20XX" or "recent myocardial infarction three weeks ago."

Subjective

- In the subjective section of the medical record, document any current complaints that are directly related to current acute myocardial infarction or old/historical myocardial infarction.

Objective

- The objective section should document any abnormal cardiovascular exam findings.
- Document the absence or presence of ST elevation on ECG/EKG tracing.

Final assessment/impression

- Document the diagnosis by spelling it out in full.
- Describe myocardial infarction with the highest level of specificity (site/location, presence or absence of ST elevation, dates/timelines).

Plan

- Document a current and specific treatment plan for acute or historical myocardial infarction, including orders for diagnostic testing.
- Document to whom/where referrals or consultation requests are made.
- Include the date of the patient's next appointment.

Myocardial infarction diagnosed on electrocardiogram or other special investigation

Many diagnostic tests, including ECG or EKG, are performed using sophisticated computer technology that includes the computer software's own diagnostic interpretation of the test results. Make sure the office note clearly documents the physician's own interpretation of test results and not simply a "cut-and-paste" of the computer software's diagnostic interpretation.

ICD-10-CM tips and resources for coders

Coding basics

There are many different ways to document and describe a myocardial infarction. ICD-10-CM code assignment is dependent upon the specific description and details documented in the individual medical record. To ensure accurate code assignment, coders must carefully review:

a) The complete medical record description of myocardial infarction

b) The alphabetic index entries and all subterms

c) The code descriptions in the tabular list, including all instructional notes

ST elevation at a glance

ST elevation myocardial infarction (STEMI) is a myocardial infarction that shows a certain change in the ECG or EKG tracing – specifically, a portion of the EKG called the ST segment is elevated above baseline.

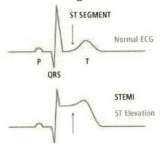

- STEMI occurs when a blood clot forms suddenly, completely blocking an artery in the heart. This can result in damage that covers a large area of the heart and extends deep into the heart muscle.

- Non-ST elevation myocardial infarction (NSTEMI) is a myocardial infarction in which the EKG tracing does NOT show elevation of the ST segment above baseline. With NSTEMI, damage does not extend through the full depth of the heart muscle.

- Note: Documentation of ST elevation on EKG by itself with no mention of acute myocardial infarction is not coded as acute myocardial infarction. Medical conditions other than acute MI can cause ST elevation. Also, for some people, ST elevation on an EKG may be a normal variant.

Coding acute myocardial infarction (AMI)

Acute myocardial infarction classifies to the following three categories:

I21   ST elevation (STEMI) and non-ST elevation (NSTEMI) myocardial infarction
Includes myocardial infarction specified as acute or with a stated duration of four weeks (28 days) or less from onset

I22   STEMI and NSTEMI myocardial infarction
Includes acute myocardial infarction occurring within four weeks (28 days) of a previous myocardial infarction, regardless of site

I23   Certain current complications following STEMI or NSTEMI myocardial infarction (within the 28-day period)

Fourth and fifth characters are required to further specify:

- ST elevation (STEMI) versus non-ST elevation (NSTEMI) myocardial infarction
- The particular site – for example, true posterior wall myocardial infarction

Acute myocardial infarction specified by site (except for subendocardial and nontransmural) but not specified as STEMI or NSTEMI should be coded to acute STEMI by site. (AHA Coding Clinic guideline for acute MI not specified as STEMI or NSTEMI, First Quarter 2013, pages 25-26)

Excerpts from the ICD-10-CM Official Guidelines for Coding and Reporting:

- If the record shows the patient was admitted with an NSTEMI that evolves to STEMI, assign the STEMI code. If STEMI converts to NSTEMI due to thrombolytic therapy, it is still coded as STEMI.

- For encounters occurring while the myocardial infarction is equal to, or less than, four weeks old, including transfers to another acute setting or a post-acute setting, and the myocardial infarction meets the definition for "other diagnoses" (see the ICD-10-CM Official Guidelines for Coding and Reporting, Section III, Reporting Additional Diagnoses), codes from category I21 may continue to be reported.

ICD-10-CM tips and resources for coders

Coding acute myocardial infarction (AMI) – continued

- For encounters after the four-week time frame during which the patient is still receiving care related to the myocardial infarction, the appropriate aftercare code should be assigned, rather than a code from category I21. For old or healed myocardial infarctions not requiring further care, code I25.2, old myocardial infarction, may be assigned.

- Code I21.3, ST elevation (STEMI) myocardial infarction of unspecified site, is the default for unspecified acute myocardial infarction. If only STEMI or transmural MI without the site is documented, assign code I21.3.

- If an AMI is documented as nontransmural or subendocardial, but the site is provided, it is still coded as a subendocardial AMI.

- A code from category I22, subsequent STEMI and NSTEMI myocardial infarction, is used when a patient who has suffered an AMI has a new AMI within the four-week time frame of the initial AMI. A code from category I22 must be used in conjunction with a code from category I21. The sequencing of the I22 and I21 codes depends on the circumstances of the encounter.

Coding old myocardial infarction

According to the ICD-10-CM manual, code I25.2 is assigned when a medical record specifically describes myocardial infarction as follows:

- Diagnosed on ECG, but presenting no symptoms
- Healed or old
- Past (diagnosed on ECG or other investigation, but currently presenting no symptoms)
- With a stated duration of four weeks or more (and no longer receiving care)
- Older than four weeks (and no longer receiving care)
- Personal history of

Diagnosed on ECG or other special investigation means the physician's own interpretation of the ECG/EKG or other diagnostic test results (and not simply a "cut-and-paste" of the diagnostic testing machine's computer software interpretation that has not been reviewed and verified by the physician).

Currently presenting no symptoms means the medical record does not document any current symptoms supported as specifically related to the old myocardial infarction.

References: American Hospital Association Coding Clinic; American College of Cardiology; ICD-10-CM Official Guidelines for Coding and Reporting; Mayo Clinic; MedlinePlus; WebMD

Clinical overview

Basic definitions

- **Neoplasm**: A new growth of tissue that serves no physiological function. A neoplasm may be:
  - **Benign** (grows in only one place; does not spread or invade other body parts but can cause problems by pressing on vital organs; does not usually recur); or
  - **Malignant** (grows, spreads and invades other body parts and can recur)
- **Cancer**: A malignant neoplasm of potentially unlimited growth that expands locally by invasion and systemically by metastasis.
- **Metastasis**: The spread of cancer from one part of the body to another. The cells of the metastatic (or secondary) cancer look like the cells of the original (or primary) cancer. Thus, pathologists can determine whether a cancer in a particular site is primary or secondary; for example, cells from a lung tumor that is a primary lung cancer look like lung cancer cells, while cells from a lung tumor that is a secondary cancer from the breast look like breast cancer cells.

For more cancer definitions, see the National Cancer Institute Dictionary of Cancer Terms at www.cancer.gov/dictionary.

Types of cancer

More than 100 different types of cancer are grouped into broader categories. The main categories are:
- Carcinoma
- Sarcoma
- Leukemia
- Lymphoma
- Myeloma
- Central nervous system cancers

Causes and risk factors for cancer

The particular cause of many cancers is unknown. Risk factors include:
- Age older than 55 (but can occur at any age)
- Lifestyle and habits (smoking, sun exposure, alcohol use, etc.)
- Family history of cancer
- Some chronic health conditions
- Environmental exposure to toxins, radiation, etc.

Signs and symptoms of cancer

Signs and symptoms of cancer depend on the type, location and stage. (Stage refers to how much the cancer has grown and spread.)

Diagnostic tools

- Medical history and physical exam
- Biopsy and pathological analysis
- Blood tests
- Diagnostic imaging (CT scans, MRI, PET scans, etc.)

Treatment

Treatment varies based on the cancer type, location and stage and may include surgical excision, chemotherapy, radiation or a combination of all three.

Documentation tips for physicians

Abbreviations

A good rule of thumb for any medical record is to limit – or avoid altogether – the use of acronyms and abbreviations. Use them only with industry-standard abbreviations. (Maintain a current list from a respected source.) Remember that some standard abbreviations have multiple meanings. The meaning of the abbreviation can often be determined based on context, but this is not always true. Best practice is as follows:

- The initial notation of a diagnosis should be spelled out in full with the abbreviation in parentheses. For example: "Prostate cancer (PCa)."
- Subsequent mention of the condition can be made using the abbreviation (PCa).
- The diagnosis should always be spelled out in full in the final impression ("prostate cancer").

Subjective

The subjective section of the office note should document the presence or absence of any current complaints or symptoms related to the neoplasm.

Objective

The objective section should include any current associated physical exam findings and results of diagnostic testing with clear dates and timelines.

Current versus historical versus remission

- Do not use the phrase "history of" to describe a current neoplasm. In diagnosis coding, "history of" means the condition is historical and no longer exists as a current problem.
- Do not use the phrase "history of" to describe a current neoplasm that is in remission. Rather, specifically describe the neoplasm as "currently in remission."

Suspected versus confirmed

- Do not use terms that imply uncertainty ("likely," probable," "apparently, "consistent with," etc.) to describe a current, confirmed neoplasm.
- Do not document a suspected and unconfirmed neoplasm as if it were confirmed. Document the signs and symptoms in the absence of a confirmed diagnosis.

Final impression

In the final diagnostic statement, describe current neoplasms to the highest level of specificity, including all of the following information:

- The histological type (adenocarcinoma, squamous cell, etc.) or behavior (benign, malignant, uncertain, unspecified)
- The exact location, including laterality and the specific site within a body part (such as inner, outer quadrant of right breast)
- Whether the neoplasm is primary, secondary or carcinoma in situ (confined to its original site with no spread)

When using the terms "metastatic" and "metastasis," clearly identify the primary and secondary sites. Consider the following examples:

Example 1	
Final diagnosis	Metastatic lung cancer
Comment	In this diagnostic statement, it is not completely clear whether the lung is the primary or secondary site.

Example 2	
Final diagnosis	Primary adenocarcinoma of the sigmoid colon with metastasis to the lung
Comment	This diagnostic statement clearly identifies the primary site (sigmoid colon) and the secondary site (lung).

Treatment plan

- Document a clear and concise plan.
- Clearly state the goal of the current plan, as in:
  - Active treatment of a current cancer; versus
  - Surveillance of a historical cancer to monitor for recurrence
- When adjuvant therapy is used, clearly state its purpose (whether the goal of adjuvant therapy is curative, palliative or preventive).
- If referrals are made or consultations requested, indicate to whom or where the referral is made or from whom consultation advice is requested.
- Document when you plan to see the patient again.

ICD-10-CM tips and resources for coders

Coding basics

For accurate and specific code assignment:
a) Review the entire medical record to verify the neoplasm is a current condition and not historical.
b) Note the exact diagnosis description documented in the medical record; then, in accordance with ICD-10-CM official coding conventions and guidelines:
c) Search the alphabetic index for that description.
d) Verify the code in the tabular list, carefully following all instructional notes.

Coding neoplasms

Most benign and all malignant neoplasms are coded from ICD-10-CM Chapter 2. Certain other benign neoplasms are found in specific body system chapters. To accurately code a current neoplasm, review the entire medical record and search for the following information regarding the neoplasm:

- Histological type (adenocarcinoma, squamous cell, etc.) or behavior (benign, malignant, uncertain)
- The exact location, including laterality if applicable, and the site within a body part (e.g., upper outer quadrant)
- Whether the neoplasm is primary, secondary or carcinoma in situ (confined to its original site with no spread)

1. If the histological type of neoplasm is documented, locate the histological term in the alphabetic index of the ICD-10-CM manual and follow the instructional notes (for example, "see also neoplasm by site, benign").
2. If the histological type is not documented, look for the neoplasm site in the neoplasm table and reference the appropriate column (malignant primary, malignant secondary, carcinoma in situ, benign, uncertain behavior, unspecified) to identify the code.
3. Then, confirm the code in the tabular list, carefully reviewing all instructional notes.

Also, review and become familiar with the ICD-10-CM Official Guidelines for Coding and Reporting for Chapter 2. These guidelines can be found in the front of the ICD-10-CM manual; the most current version for each year can be found on the website of the Centers for Disease Control and Prevention (CDC). Be sure to use the official guidelines that cover the date of service being coded.

Unspecified cancer site

- Code C80.0, disseminated malignant neoplasm, unspecified, is assigned only in those cases in which the patient has advanced metastatic disease and no known primary or secondary sites are specified. It should not be used in place of assigning codes for the primary site and all known secondary sites.
- Code C80.1, malignant (primary) neoplasm, unspecified, is assigned only when no determination can be made as to the primary site of a malignancy.
- Code C79.9, secondary malignant neoplasm of unspecified site, is assigned when no site is specified for the secondary neoplasm.
- When no site is indicated in the diagnostic statement but the morphology type is stated as metastatic, the code provided for that morphological type is assigned for the primary diagnosis along with an additional code for secondary neoplasm of unspecified site.

Example	
Diagnosis	Metastatic apocrine adenocarcinoma
ICD-10-CM codes	This diagnosis is coded as a primary malignant neoplasm of the skin, site unspecified – C44.99 plus code C79.9 for the unspecified secondary site.
Rationale	Code C44.99 is obtained by referring to the main term "adenocarcinoma" followed by subterms "apocrine" and "unspecified site."

Primary versus secondary site

The terms "metastatic" and "metastasis" are often used ambiguously in describing neoplasms, sometimes meaning that the site named is primary and sometimes meaning it is secondary. When the diagnostic statement is not clear in this regard, the coder should review the medical record for further information. When none is available, however, the following guidelines apply.

- **"Metastatic to"** means the site mentioned is secondary. For example, "metastatic carcinoma to the lung" is coded as secondary malignant neoplasm of the lung (C78.0-).
- **"Metastatic from"** means the site mentioned is the primary site. For example, "metastatic carcinoma from the breast" indicates the breast is the primary site (C50.9-). An additional code for the metastatic site also should be assigned.

ICD-10-CM tips and resources for coders

Primary versus secondary site – continued

- **Multiple metastatic sites** – When two or more sites are described in the diagnosis as "metastatic," each of the stated sites should be coded as secondary or metastatic. A code also should be assigned for the primary site when this information is available; it should be coded as C80.1 when it is not.

- **Single metastatic site** – When only one site is described as metastatic without any further qualification and no more definitive information can be obtained by reviewing the medical record, the following steps should be used:

Step 1

- Refer first to the morphology type in the alphabetic index and code to the primary condition of that site. For example, "metastatic renal cell carcinoma of the lung" indicates the primary site is the kidney (C64.9) and the secondary site is the lung (C78.00).

- When a specific site for morphology type is not indicated in a code entry or not indexed, assign the code for unspecified site within that anatomical site. For example, "oat cell carcinoma" codes to C34.90, malignant neoplasm of unspecified part of unspecified bronchus or lung, when no more specific site is stated.

Step 2

- When the morphology type is not stated or the only code that can be obtained is either C80.0 or C80.1, code as a primary malignant neoplasm, unless the site is one of the following:

• bone	• liver	• peritoneum
• brain	• lymph nodes	• pleura
• diaphragm	• mediastinum	• retroperitoneum
• heart	• meninges	• spinal cord

- Sites classifiable to category C76, malignant neoplasms of other and ill-defined sites

Malignant neoplasms of these sites are coded as secondary sites when not otherwise specified, except neoplasm of the liver, for which ICD-10-CM provides the following code: C22.9, malignant neoplasm of liver, not specified as primary or secondary.

Diagnosis	Metastatic carcinoma of the lung
ICD-10-CM codes	Lung is not in the list under Step 2; therefore, the lung is coded as the primary site (C34.90) with the secondary site unknown (C79.9).

Diagnosis	Metastatic bone cancer
ICD-10-CM codes	Bone is in the list under Step 2; therefore, bone is coded as secondary (C79.51) with the primary site unknown (C80.1).

Diagnosis	Metastatic prostate cancer
ICD-10-CM codes	The prostate is not in the list under Step 2; therefore, the prostate is coded as the primary site (C61) with the secondary site unknown (C79.9).

Coding cancer as current

Generally, cancer is coded as current when the medical record clearly shows active treatment directed to the cancer for the purpose of cure or palliation and/or when the record clearly shows the cancer is present but:

a) It is unresponsive to treatment;

b) The current treatment plan is watchful waiting or observation only; or

c) The patient has refused any further treatment.

Active cancer treatment can include adjuvant therapy for cure or palliation. Adjuvant therapy (any treatment given after the primary therapy to increase the chance of long-term disease-free survival) may include chemotherapy, radiation therapy, hormone therapy, targeted therapy or biological therapy.

Coding cancer in remission

The National Cancer Institute defines "remission" as:

A decrease in or disappearance of signs and symptoms of cancer. In partial remission, some, but not all, signs and symptoms of cancer have disappeared. In complete remission, all signs and symptoms of cancer have disappeared, although cancer still may be in the body.

When coding a cancer described in the final diagnosis as currently in remission, carefully review the entire record to determine whether overall context supports coding the cancer in remission as a current, active condition versus a historical condition. For example, look for documentation of unrealistic time frames that indicate a historical diagnosis (for example, cancer in remission noted as eradicated many years ago with no current treatment and no documented evidence of current cancer should be coded as historical).

ICD-10-CM tips and resources for coders

Coding lymphoma

The Lymphoma Research Foundation advises as follows: Lymphoma – the most common blood cancer – has two main forms: Hodgkin lymphoma and non-Hodgkin lymphoma. Lymphoma occurs when cells of the immune system called lymphocytes, a type of white blood cell, grow and multiply uncontrollably. Cancerous lymphocytes can travel to many parts of the body – including the lymph nodes, spleen, bone marrow, blood or other organs – and form a tumor. The body has two main types of lymphocytes that can develop into lymphomas: B-lymphocytes (B-cells) and T-lymphocytes (T-cells).

- ICD-10-CM has many categories and subcategories for lymphomas with fourth and fifth characters that provide further specificity, including the particular type of lymphoma and the affected sites.
- Lymphomas can be malignant or benign. Benign lymphomas classify to code D36.Ø, benign neoplasm of lymph nodes.
- Malignant lymphomas classify to the following categories:

Hodgkin lymphoma	Non-Hodgkin lymphoma
C81	C82, C83, C84, C85, C86, C88

- Lymphomas are systemic diseases that do not metastasize in the same way as solid tumors, which are not lymphomas. A lymphoma, regardless of the number of sites involved, is not considered metastatic and is never coded as secondary cancer.
- Lymphoma patients in remission are still considered to have lymphoma, and the appropriate ICD-10-CM code representing current lymphoma should be assigned.

Coding historical cancer

A primary malignancy is coded as historical (category Z85, personal history of malignant neoplasm) after the primary malignancy has been excised or eradicated, there is no further treatment directed to that site and there is no current evidence of any existing primary malignancy.

Encounter for follow-up examination after treatment for malignant neoplasm has been completed is coded as ZØ8. This code includes medical surveillance following completed treatment (i.e., monitoring for cancer recurrence) and *Excludes1* aftercare following medical care (Z43–Z49, Z51). Code ZØ8 advises to use an additional code to identify any acquired absence of organs (Z9Ø.-) and personal history of malignant neoplasm (Z85.-).

References: American Hospital Association Coding Clinic; ICD-10-CM and ICD-10-PCS Coding Handbook; ICD-10-CM Official Guidelines for Coding and Reporting; Lymphoma Research Foundation; Mayo Clinic; MedlinePlus; National Cancer Institute

Morbid Obesity/Body Mass Index (BMI)   ICD-10-CM

Clinical overview

Definitions and background

- **Centers for Disease Control and Prevention (CDC):** Overweight and obesity are labels for ranges of weight that are greater than what is generally considered healthy for a given height. The terms also identify ranges of weight that have been shown to increase the likelihood of certain diseases and other health problems.

- **MedlinePlus** (a service of the U.S. National Library of Medicine and the National Institutes of Health, or NIH): "Obesity means having too much body fat. It is different from being overweight, which means weighing too much. The weight may come from muscle, bone, fat and/or body water. Both terms mean that a person's weight is greater than what's considered healthy for his or her height."

- **The NIH** definition of morbid obesity:
  - Being 100 pounds or more above ideal body weight; or
  - Having a BMI of 40 or greater; or
  - Having a BMI of 35 or greater and one or more comorbid conditions

- **The National Heart, Lung and Blood Institute (NHLBI):** Assessment of an obese patient should include evaluation of BMI, waist circumference and overall medical risk. NHLBI uses the terms "clinically severe obesity" and "extreme obesity" in place of the commonly used term "morbid obesity."

	Body mass index	Obesity class
Underweight	< 18.5	
Normal	18.5 – 24.9	
Overweight	25.0 – 29.9	
Obesity	30.0 – 34.9	1
	35.0 – 39.9	2
Extreme obesity	$\geq$ 40	3

- The preferred obesity metric in research is body fat percentage (BF%) – the ratio of the total weight of a person's fat to his or her body weight. Accurate measurement of BF% is much more difficult than BMI* measurement; BMI can be used to approximate BF%.

BMI*

BMI is a mathematical calculation – a person's weight in kilograms divided by height in meters squared. Although BMI correlates with the amount of body fat, BMI does not directly measure body fat. Thus, some people (athletes, for example) may have a BMI identifying them as overweight even though they do not have excess body fat.

- Other methods to measure body fatness include underwater weighing, bioelectrical impedance, dual-energy X-ray absorptiometry and isotope dilution. However, these methods are not always readily available, they can be expensive, they need to be conducted by highly trained personnel, and they can be difficult to standardize across observers or machines, complicating comparisons across studies and time periods.

In general, BMI is an inexpensive and easy-to-perform method of screening for obesity/morbid obesity. Even though a high BMI can be an indicator of high body fatness, calculation of BMI is only a screening tool; it is not diagnostic of the body fatness or health of an individual.

The correlation between BMI and body fatness is fairly strong, but even if two people have the same BMI, their levels of body fatness may differ.

To determine if a high BMI is a health risk for an individual person, a physician would perform further assessments (such as those methods noted above), as well as evaluations of diet, physical activity, personal history including comorbidities, family history and other appropriate health screenings.

Summary: Physicians use multiple resources and criteria to define and diagnose obesity-related conditions. BMI is a screening tool only. It is not the only criterion used to diagnose obesity/morbid obesity. Diagnosis code assignment is based on the physician's clinical judgment and corresponding medical record description of the specific obesity condition.

Clinical overview – continued

Causes and risk factors for development of obesity

- Physical inactivity
- Unhealthy diet
- Unhealthy eating habits
- Lack of adequate sleep
- Certain medications
- Certain medical conditions
- Genetics and family history
- Older age
- Social and economic issues
- Cultural issues

Signs and symptoms

- Clothes feeling tight/need for larger-size clothing
- Increased weight and BMI
- Increased waist circumference

Diagnostic tools

- Medical history and physical exam
- Calculation of height, weight and BMI
- Measurement of body fat percentage
- Measurement of waist circumference
- Evaluation of comorbid conditions

Complications and health risks

Short-term

- Shortness of breath with activity and exertion
- Difficulty sleeping
- Snoring
- Fatigue
- Back and joint pain

Long-term

- High blood pressure and hypertension
- High cholesterol and triglycerides
- Type 2 diabetes mellitus
- Metabolic syndrome
- Heart disease
- Stroke
- Kidney disease
- Sleep apnea
- Cancer
- Fatty liver disease
- Gallbladder disease
- Osteoarthritis

Medical treatment

- Medications
- Weight-loss surgery

Prevention and self-management

- Nutritionally balanced diet
- Healthy eating habits, including portion control
- Regular physical exercise
- Good sleep habits
- Tracking and trending weight, BMI and waist circumference
- Behavior modification
- Support groups
- Realistic goal setting

Morbid Obesity/Body Mass Index (BMI)   ICD-10-CM

Documentation tips for physicians

Subjective

- Document the presence or absence of any current symptoms related to obesity, morbid obesity, overweight, etc.

Objective

- Document the patient's height, weight and BMI. (The medical coder is not allowed to use the patient's documented height and weight to calculate the BMI and assign a corresponding ICD-10-CM code. Rather, the medical record must specifically document the BMI.)
- In the physical exam, document with the highest specificity any current associated observations or findings (such as overweight, obese, morbidly obese, etc.).

Final assessment/impression

- Document the overweight or obesity diagnosis with the highest level of specificity, as in "morbid obesity," "severe obesity," "extreme obesity," etc.
- Include any associated diagnoses that caused the overweight or obesity condition.
  - Use terms that clearly show the cause-and-effect relationship (such as "due to," "secondary to," "related to," etc.).
- Include any coexisting diagnoses that are impacted by the overweight or obesity diagnosis.
- Do not describe a current obesity diagnosis as "history of."

Plan

- Document a clear and concise treatment plan (e.g., referral to nutritionist; patient education related to the obesity condition with information regarding balanced diet; plan for return follow-up; etc.).

ICD-10-CM tips and resources for coders

Coding obesity

Overweight and obesity classify to subcategory E66 as follows:

E66.Ø- Obesity due to excess calories

    E66.Ø1 Morbid (severe) obesity due to excess calories

    E66.Ø9 Other obesity due to excess calories

E66.1 Drug-induced obesity

E66.2 Morbid (severe) obesity with alveolar hypoventilation

E66.3 Overweight

E66.8 Other obesity

E66.9 Obesity, unspecified

Use an additional code to identify BMI if known (Z68).

Coding BMI – category Z68

- Adult BMI codes are used for persons 21 years of age or older and classify as follows:

Code

Z68.1 Body mass index [BMI] 19 or less, adult

Subcategories

Z68.2 Body mass index [BMI] 20-29.9, adult

Z68.3 Body mass index [BMI] 30-39.9, adult

Z68.4 Body mass index [BMI] 40 or greater, adult

Fifth characters are added to identify the specific BMI range within subcategories Z68.2 – Z68.4.

Clinical significance of BMI

- BMI codes are reported only as secondary diagnoses in association with a primary diagnosis for which the BMI has clinical significance. As with all other secondary diagnosis codes, the BMI codes are assigned only when they meet the definition of a reportable additional diagnosis (per ICD-10-CM Official Guidelines for Coding and Reporting).
  - Primary diagnoses for which BMI has clinical significance would be any primary condition that can be either:
    - a) improved if the patient loses weight or lowers his/her BMI; or
    - b) worsened if the patient gains weight or increases his/her BMI.

Examples include but are not limited to: Diabetes mellitus, hypertension, hyperlipidemia, obstructive sleep apnea

Additional tips and reminders for coding BMI

Code assignment for BMI may be based on medical record documentation from clinicians who are not the patient's provider (i.e., physician or other qualified health care practitioner legally accountable for establishing the patient's diagnosis), since this information is typically documented by other clinicians involved in the care of the patient (e.g., a dietitian often documents BMI).

- However, the associated diagnosis (such as overweight or obesity) must be documented by the patient's provider. If there is conflicting medical record documentation, either from the same clinician or different clinicians, the patient's attending provider should be queried for clarification.

Reminder: Physicians use multiple resources and criteria to define and diagnose obesity-related conditions. BMI is a screening tool only; it is not the only criterion used to diagnose obesity/morbid obesity. Diagnosis code assignment is based on the physician's clinical judgment and corresponding medical record description of the specific obesity condition.

References: American Hospital Association Coding Clinic; American Heart Association; Centers for Disease Control and Prevention; Cleveland Clinic; ICD-10-CM Official Guidelines for Coding and Reporting; Mayo Clinic; MedlinePlus; National Heart, Lung and Blood Institute; National Institute of Diabetes and Digestive and Kidney Diseases; National Institute of Health

Clinical overview

Definitions

"Peripheral vascular disease" is a broad term that refers to diseases of the blood vessels outside the heart and brain. These diseases, over time, cause occlusion of the peripheral blood vessels by the following mechanisms:

- Inflammation: narrowing of blood vessels
- Atherosclerosis (fatty deposits): blockage of blood vessels
- Thrombus (clot) formation: blockage of blood vessels

Occlusion of the peripheral blood vessels results in restriction of blood flow.

Peripheral venous (vein) disease

The most common type of peripheral venous disease is deep vein thrombosis (DVT), or clot. See the separate DVT coding guidelines.

Peripheral arterial (artery) disease (PAD)

This guideline focuses on the most common type of peripheral vascular disease: peripheral arterial disease.

- PAD is most commonly caused by atherosclerosis or "hardening of the arteries." This problem occurs when fatty material (plaque) builds up along the walls of the arteries (similar to coronary artery disease), causing narrowing of the arteries that reduces blood flow. In addition, the arterial walls become stiffer and cannot widen (dilate) properly, which also interferes with normal blood flow.
- People with PAD often also have coronary artery disease (CAD) and thus have a higher risk of heart attack or stroke. PAD mainly affects the arteries of the arms, legs, kidneys and stomach, but it usually begins in the legs.

Risk factors

- Atherosclerosis
- Diabetes mellitus
- Smoking
- Abnormal cholesterol levels
- Hyperlipidemia
- Heart disease
- High blood pressure/hypertension
- Obesity
- Older age
- Family history of PAD

Signs and symptoms (usually affect lower extremities)

- Most common symptom of PAD is intermittent claudication (pain or discomfort in the lower extremities and buttocks that occurs with exercise/activity and resolves with rest)
- Diminished pulses in legs or feet
- Decreased blood pressure in the affected limb(s)
- Arterial bruits (a whooshing sound heard with a stethoscope over the artery)
- Ulceration and sores with poor healing
- Hair loss on the legs and feet
- Discoloration of skin (bluish, dusky)
- Decreased warmth in the lower extremities

Diagnostic tools

- Medical history and physical exam
- Ankle-brachial index (ABI) test (compares blood pressures of the ankle and arm)
- Laboratory testing (e.g., blood testing for elevated cholesterol or diabetes)
- Ultrasound of the lower extremities
- Angiography of the arteries of the lower extremities

Complications

- Ulcers or open sores in or on legs and feet that can become infected and can lead to amputation
- Increased risk for heart attack and stroke

Treatment

- Smoking cessation
- Management of underlying conditions such as diabetes, high cholesterol and high blood pressure
- Diet management, exercise and weight control
- Medications (to prevent blood clots, to control pain if needed, to improve blood flow, etc.)
- Surgery (e.g., angioplasty)

Documentation tips for physicians

Abbreviations

- Limit – or avoid altogether – the use of acronyms and abbreviations. The abbreviation PVD is sometimes used to refer to peripheral vascular disease; however, PVD can have other meanings (e.g., posterior vitreous detachment, portal vein dilation). Further, in handwritten office notes, "PVD" is sometimes misinterpreted as "PUD" (e.g., peptic ulcer disease).
- The meaning of an abbreviation can often be determined based on context, but this is not always true.
- Further, "peripheral vascular disease" is a broad, nonspecific diagnosis.
- Best practice is to clearly spell out and fully describe the particular type of peripheral vascular disease that is present and all related manifestations.

Subjective

- In the subjective section of the medical record, document the presence or absence of any current symptoms related to peripheral vascular disease (e.g., pain, cold extremities, etc.).
- When intermittent claudication is present, clearly describe the patient's particular symptoms.

Objective

- The objective section should document any current associated physical exam findings (diminished pulses, hair loss, skin discoloration, etc.) and related diagnostic testing results.

Final assessment/impression

- The final diagnostic statement should spell out in full and clearly describe the particular type of peripheral vascular disease condition that is present.
  - Document the site/location.
  - Specify the underlying causative condition and any related manifestations by using appropriate descriptors and/or linking terms such as "due to," "secondary to," "associated with," "related to," etc.
    Example: "Atherosclerotic peripheral vascular disease of bilateral lower extremities with intermittent claudication"

Final assessment/impression – continued

- When documenting occlusive peripheral arterial disease, specify the cause of the occlusion.
- Do not describe current peripheral vascular disease as "history of." In diagnosis coding, the phrase "history of" means the condition is historical and no longer exists as a current problem.
- Do not include a past peripheral vascular condition that has resolved as if it is current.
- Do not use terms that imply uncertainty ("probable," "apparently," "likely," "consistent with," etc.) to describe a current, confirmed peripheral vascular disease condition.
- Do not document suspected and unconfirmed peripheral vascular disease as if it were confirmed. Document signs and symptoms in the absence of a confirmed diagnosis.
- Include the current status of the peripheral vascular disease condition (stable, improved, worsening, etc.).

Plan

- Document a clear and specific treatment plan for the PVD condition, including orders for future diagnostic testing.
- Document to whom/where referrals or consultation requests are made.
- Include the date of the patient's next appointment.

Electronic medical record (EMR) reminder

- Some electronic medical records insert ICD-10-CM code descriptions into the medical record to represent the final diagnosis, for example: "I73.89 Other specified peripheral vascular disease."
  - Remember that with these types of vague descriptions the diagnosis will not be complete unless the physician clearly documents the specific "other" PVD.

ICD-10-CM tips and resources for coders

Coding basics

Many different descriptors further specify the particular types of peripheral vascular disease. For accurate and specific diagnosis code assignment, the coder must:

a) Review the entire medical record to verify the PVD condition is current.

b) Note the exact PVD description documented in the medical record; then, in accordance with ICD-10-CM official coding conventions and guidelines:

c) Search the alphabetic index for that specific description.

d) Verify the code in the tabular list, carefully following all instructional notes.

Coding PVD

- Vague diagnoses, such as "peripheral vascular disease" or "intermittent claudication" without further specification, should be clarified with the physician. However, when physician query is not possible and the medical record clearly supports a current diagnosis stated simply as "peripheral vascular disease," the code that must be assigned is I73.9, peripheral vascular disease, unspecified. This code includes:
  - ○ Intermittent claudication
  - ○ Peripheral angiopathy not otherwise specified
  - ○ Spasm of artery

Abbreviation PVD

A common coding error involves misinterpretation of the abbreviation PVD, especially in handwritten notes (for example, PUD for peptic ulcer disease can easily be misread as PVD). Further, the abbreviation PVD can have other meanings. Use caution when coding PVD – code I73.9 should not be assigned unless the individual medical record clearly shows PVD is being used to represent peripheral vascular disease.

Atherosclerosis of the native arteries of the extremities

Atherosclerosis of the native arteries of the extremities classifies to subcategory I70.2-. An additional code is used, if applicable, to identify chronic total occlusion of artery of extremity (I70.92).

Fifth characters in subcategory I70.2- specify the progression of the disease as follows:

I70.20-	Unspecified atherosclerosis of native arteries of extremities
I70.21-	Atherosclerosis of native arteries of extremities with intermittent claudication
I70.22-	Atherosclerosis of native arteries of extremities with rest pain (includes any intermittent claudication)
I70.23- I70.24- I70.25-	Atherosclerosis of native arteries of extremities with ulceration (includes any rest pain and/or intermittent claudication) Code L97.- is used with I70.23- and I70.24-, and code L98.49- is used with I70.25-, to identify the severity of the ulcer.
I70.26-	Atherosclerosis of native arteries of extremities with gangrene (includes any or all of the preceding conditions). I70.26- advises to use an additional code to identify the severity of any ulcer (L97.-, L98.49), if applicable.

As noted, these codes are listed in order of priority, and the codes are hierarchical, meaning the higher-level codes include the conditions of the lower-level codes. For example, if the patient has atherosclerosis of native arteries with ulceration and gangrene, only a code from subcategory I70.26- is assigned, as this code includes both gangrene and ulceration.

ICD-10-CM tips and resources for coders

Atherosclerosis of extremities involving a graft

Atherosclerosis of extremities involving a graft codes to I7Ø.3- through I7Ø.7-, as follows:

I7Ø.3-	Atherosclerosis of unspecified type of bypass graft(s) of the extremities
I7Ø.4-	Atherosclerosis of autologous vein bypass graft(s) of the extremities
I7Ø.5-	Atherosclerosis of nonautologous biological bypass graft(s) of the extremities
I7Ø.6-	Atherosclerosis of nonbiological bypass graft(s) of the extremities.
I7Ø.7-	Atherosclerosis of other type of bypass graft(s) of the extremities.

Codes from I7Ø.3- through I7Ø.7- provide additional characters to indicate the same progression of disease discussed above under subcategory I7Ø.2 – namely, intermittent claudication, rest pain, ulceration and gangrene.

- A chronic total occlusion of an artery of the extremities (I7Ø.92) develops when hard, calcified plaque accumulates in an artery over an extended period of time, resulting in a clinically significant decrease in blood flow. Approximately 40 percent of patients with peripheral vascular disease present initially with partial occlusion, which progresses to a chronic total occlusion. Intervention with angioplasty and stenting is more complex because passing a guide wire through a total occlusion is extremely difficult.
- Code I7Ø.92 is assigned as an additional code with subcategories I7Ø.3- through I7Ø.7- when a chronic total occlusion is present with atherosclerosis of the extremities.

Diabetic vascular disease

Peripheral vascular disease is a frequent complication of diabetes mellitus.

- Diabetic peripheral vascular disease without gangrene codes to EØ8 – E13 with .51.
- Diabetic peripheral vascular disease with gangrene codes to EØ8 – E13 with .52.
- Diabetes with other circulatory complications codes to EØ8 – E13 with .59.

Although atherosclerosis may occur earlier and more extensively in patients with diabetes, coronary artery disease, cardiomyopathy and cerebrovascular disease are not complications of diabetes and are not included in subcategories EØ8 – E13 with .5-.

- These conditions are coded separately unless the physician documents a causal relationship.

Further, the blood vessels of the heart and brain are not part of the peripheral circulatory system. Thus, when atherosclerotic heart or brain disease is linked in the record to diabetes mellitus as the cause, they are not coded as peripheral vascular diseases. Rather, these types of diabetic vascular complications are coded to EØ8 – E13 with .59.

References: American Hospital Association (AHA) Coding Clinic; American College of Cardiology; ICD-10-CM Official Guidelines for Coding and Reporting; ICD-10-CM and ICD-10-PCS Coding Handbook; Mayo Clinic; MedlinePlus; WebMD

Pressure Injury (formerly Pressure Ulcer) ICD-10-CM

Clinical overview

Background and NPUAP terminology/definition

In April 2016, the National Pressure Ulcer Advisory Panel (NPUAP) announced a change in terminology from "pressure ulcer" to "pressure injury" and also updated the stages of pressure injury. The change in terminology more accurately describes pressure injuries to both intact and ulcerated skin.

A pressure injury is localized damage to the skin and underlying soft tissue, usually over a bony prominence or related to a medical or other device. The injury can present as intact skin or an open ulcer and may be painful. The injury occurs as a result of intense and/or prolonged pressure or pressure in combination with shear. The tolerance of soft tissue for pressure and shear may also be affected by microclimate, nutrition, perfusion, comorbidities and condition of the soft tissue.

Causes and risk factors

- Immobility (being bedridden or requiring the use of a wheelchair; being unable to change position without help – e.g., post-surgery, due to coma or paralysis)
- Fragile skin
- Moisture (such as with incontinence of bowel or bladder or excessive perspiration)
- Poor nutrition
- Mental disability that interferes with ability to prevent or treat pressure ulcers
- Older age
- Poorly fitting prosthetic devices
- Chronic conditions that cause poor circulation or lack of pain perception
- Smoking (nicotine impairs circulation)

Complications

- Bone and joint infections
- Cellulitis
- Sepsis
- Skin cancer

Diagnostic tools

- Medical history and physical exam
- Skin or wound culture if infection is suspected
- Skin biopsy
- Diagnostic testing related to underlying contributing conditions and to evaluate nutritional status

Signs and symptoms

The NPUAP provides detailed descriptions and illustrations of the signs and symptoms associated with each stage of pressure injury:

- **Stage 1: Nonblanchable erythema of intact skin**
- **Stage 2: Partial-thickness skin loss with exposed dermis**
- **Stage 3: Full-thickness skin loss**
- **Stage 4: Full-thickness skin and tissue loss**
- **Unstageable pressure injury: Obscured full-thickness skin and tissue loss**
- **Deep-tissue pressure injury: Persistent nonblanchable deep red, maroon or purple discoloration**
  http://www.npuap.org/resources/educational-and-clinical-resources/npuap-pressure-injury-stages/

Pressure injury staging illustrations

http://www.npuap.org/resources/educational-and-clinical-resources/pressure-injury-staging-illustrations/

Prevention

- Regular and frequent skin inspection to monitor for early signs and symptoms of pressure injury
- Proper positioning with frequent position changes
- Proper skin care (keeping skin clean and moisturized, but avoiding too much moisture)
- Balanced nutrition
- Avoidance of sliding or dragging maneuvers
- Smoking cessation
- Exercise
- Individual and caregiver education

Treatment

- Implementation of preventive measures, such as those listed above
- Relieving pressure on the area (devices such as foam pads or air-filled mattresses may be used)
- Pain and infection management
- Management and treatment of contributing underlying conditions
- Other treatment based on the stage of the pressure ulcer and according to physician orders, which may include cleaning the ulcer, dressing changes, ointments, creams, medications, debridement procedures and surgery

Pressure Injury (formerly Pressure Ulcer) ICD-10-CM

Documentation tips for physicians

Abbreviations
A good rule of thumb for any medical record is to limit – or avoid altogether – the use of abbreviations. Best practice is to spell out "pressure ulcer" or "pressure injury" in full, along with a detailed description.

Subjective
The subjective section of the office note should document any current patient or caregiver complaint related to pressure injury.

Objective
The objective section of the office note should document the physical examination findings and detailed description of any current pressure ulcer, including the following:

- The specific site/location, including laterality
- The specific stage (per NPUAP descriptions)
- Precise measurements (length, width, depth in centimeters)
- Undermining, sinus tracts or tunneling (recorded in centimeters)
- Wound-base description (granulation, necrotic tissue, eschar, slough, new epithelial tissue)
- Absence or presence of drainage (amount, color, consistency and odor as appropriate)
- Wound edges – description of area up to 4 cm from edge of the wound; measure in centimeters and describe characteristics (light pink, deep red, purple, macerated, calloused, etc.)
- Odor – present or absent
- Any associated pain and related intervention
- Current status (improved, no change, stable, etc.)

Final assessment/impression
- Do not describe a current pressure ulcer as "history of." In diagnosis coding, the phrase "history of" means the condition is historical and no longer exists as a current problem.
- Do not document a past pressure ulcer that has resolved as if it were current.
- Document the current status of pressure ulcers (stable, no change, improved, worsening, etc.), and refer the reader back to the physical exam description.

Treatment plan
Document a specific and concise treatment plan for pressure ulcers (e.g., devices such as foam pads or mattresses; wound care instructions; prescriptions for ointments, creams or other medications; planned debridement; etc.).

- If referrals are made or consultations requested, the office note should indicate to whom or where the referral or consultation is made or from whom consultation advice is requested.
- Document when the patient will be seen again.

Documentation and coding examples

Example 1	
Final diagnosis	1.0 cm decubitus ulcer sacral region
ICD-10-CM code	**L89.159** Pressure ulcer of sacral region, unspecified stage

Example 2	
Final diagnosis	Stage 4 gangrenous pressure ulcer right heel
ICD-10-CM codes	**I96** Gangrene, not elsewhere classified **L89.614** Pressure ulcer of right heel, stage 4

Example 3	
Final diagnosis	Pressure ulcer left lower back, not staged since covered with dressing and patient refused to have it removed and redressed.
ICD-10-CM code	**L89.140** Pressure ulcer of left lower back, unstageable

Example 4	
Final diagnosis	Stage 1 right foot ulcer
ICD-10-CM code	**L97.519** Nonpressure chronic ulcer of other part of right foot with unspecified severity

ICD-10-CM tips and resources for coders

Coding basics

For accurate and specific diagnosis code assignment, the coder must:

- Review the entire medical record to verify pressure ulcer/pressure injury is a current condition.
- Note the exact description of the pressure injury documented in the medical record; then, according to ICD-10-CM official coding conventions and guidelines:
  a) Search the alphabetic index for that specific description.
  b) Verify the code in the tabular list, carefully following all instructional notes.

Coding pressure ulcers

The ICD-10-CM Official Guidelines for Coding and Reporting (Section I.C.12.a.1-6) provides detailed information regarding coding of pressure ulcer stages.

1) **Pressure ulcer stages**
   - Codes in category L89, pressure ulcer, are combination codes that identify the site and stage of the pressure ulcer.

     Fifth characters identify the specific site of the ulcer – e.g., elbow (L89.0-); back (L89.1-); hip (L89.2-); buttock (L89.3-); contiguous site of back, buttock and hip (L89.4-); ankle (L89.5-); heel (L89.6-); other site (L89.8-); and unspecified site (L89.9-).

     The sixth character indicates the severity of the ulcer by identifying the stage. ICD-10-CM classifies pressure ulcer stages based on severity designated by stages 1-4, unspecified stage and unstageable.

   - Assign as many codes from category L89 as needed to identify all the pressure ulcers the patient has, if applicable.

2) **Unstageable pressure ulcers**
   - Assignment of the code for unstageable pressure ulcer (L89.--0) should be based on the clinical documentation. These codes are used for:
     - Pressure ulcers of which the stage cannot be clinically determined (e.g., the ulcer is covered by eschar or has been treated with a skin or muscle graft)
     - Pressure ulcers that are documented as deep-tissue injury but not documented as due to trauma
   - This code should not be confused with the codes for unspecified stage (L89.--9), which are used when there is no documentation regarding the stage of the pressure ulcer.

3) **Documented pressure ulcer stage**
   - Assignment of the code for the pressure ulcer stage should be guided by clinical documentation of the stage or documentation of the terms found in the alphabetic index.
   - For clinical terms describing the stage that are not found in the alphabetic index, and for which there is no documentation of the stage, the physician or other health care provider should be queried.

4) **Pressure ulcers documented as healed**
   - No code is assigned if the documentation states the pressure ulcer is completely healed.

5) **Pressure ulcers documented as healing**
   - For pressure ulcers described as healing, assign the appropriate pressure ulcer stage code based on the documentation in the medical record. If the documentation does not provide information about the stage of the healing pressure ulcer, assign the appropriate code for unspecified stage.
   - If the documentation is unclear as to whether the patient has a current (new) pressure ulcer or if the patient is being treated for a healing pressure ulcer, query the physician or other health care provider.
   - For ulcers that were present on (inpatient) admission but healed at the time of discharge, assign the code for the site and stage of the pressure ulcer at the time of admission.

6) **Patient admitted with pressure ulcer evolving into another stage during the admission**
   - If a patient is admitted with a pressure ulcer at one stage and it progresses to a higher stage, two separate codes should be assigned:
     a) One code for the site and stage of the ulcer on admission; and
     b) A second code for the same ulcer site and the highest stage reported during the stay.

Pressure Injury (formerly Pressure Ulcer) ICD-10-CM

ICD-10-CM tips and resources for coders

Coding pressure injury

As noted in the clinical overview section, in April 2016, the National Pressure Ulcer Advisory Panel (NPUAP) announced a change in terminology from "pressure ulcer" to "pressure injury" and also updated the stages of pressure injury. The change in terminology more accurately describes pressure injuries to both intact and ulcerated skin.

Please note: This is a change in terminology, not a change in the definition of pressure ulcer.

- For pressure injury meaning pressure ulcer, code as a pressure ulcer by the site and stage or unstageable, as appropriate.
- The stages of pressure injury used in the NPUAP's updated terminology correspond to the pressure ulcer stages in ICD-10-CM. Therefore, code a non-traumatic pressure injury the same as a pressure ulcer by site with stages 1 through 4 and unstageable.
  - For example, pressure injury, stages 1-4, is coded as pressure ulcer, stages 1-4.
  - A deep-tissue injury is coded as an unstageable pressure ulcer. In ICD-10-CM, there is an existing index entry under deep-tissue injury:

    Injury
       deep tissue
          meaning pressure ulcer – *see* Ulcer pressure, unstageable, by site

Classifications and staging of diabetic foot ulcers

There are classification systems that grade or stage diabetic foot ulcers from no ulcer to superficial ulcer to deep/infected/ischemic or gangrenous ulcers. Examples include the Wagner system or the University of Texas system.

- These classification systems should not be confused with pressure ulcer staging. A staged diabetic foot ulcer is not coded as a pressure ulcer unless the medical record clearly states the diabetic foot ulcer is a pressure ulcer.

Staged ulcers not described as pressure ulcers

The fact that an ulcer is staged does not, by itself, support coding as a pressure ulcer. For a staged ulcer to be coded as a pressure ulcer, the staged ulcer must be described with terms that classify to pressure ulcer (e.g., pressure ulcer, pressure injury, decubitus ulcer, bed sore, etc.).

References: American Hospital Association Coding Clinic; ICD-10-CM and ICD-10-PCS Coding Handbook; ICD-10-CM Official Guidelines for Coding and Reporting; Mayo Clinic; MedlinePlus; Merck Manual; National Pressure Ulcer Advisory Panel

Clinical overview

American Cancer Society and other resources

- The American Cancer Society website provides in-depth information about prostate cancer, including but not limited to, causes, risk factors and prevention; early detection, diagnosis and staging; and treatment. https://www.cancer.org/cancer/prostate-cancer.html
- There are many other respected sources for prostate cancer information. See the references section on the next page of this guideline.

Prostate-specific antigen (PSA)

PSA is a protein produced by cells of the prostate gland that often is elevated in men with prostate cancer. The PSA laboratory test measures the level of PSA in a man's blood. PSA testing often is used with a digital rectal examination of the prostate gland to screen for prostate cancer. Other noncancerous conditions, however, can cause an elevated PSA – for example, inflammation or enlargement of the prostate gland.

Generally, a PSA level of 4.0 ng/mL or less is considered normal. Recent studies have shown, however, that some men with PSA levels below 4.0 have prostate cancer, while other men with higher levels do not have prostate cancer. There are various causes of fluctuations in PSA levels, but generally the higher the PSA level, the more likely the diagnosis of prostate cancer. A continuous rise in PSA level over time may be a sign of prostate cancer.

Prostate cancer treatment

- Watchful waiting and active surveillance
- Surgical removal of the prostate (prostatectomy)
- Cryosurgery (freezing cancer cells with cold metal probes)
- Chemotherapy
- Hormonal therapy
- External radiation
- Internal radiation (radioactive seed implantation)

Hormone therapy for prostate cancer

Most prostate cancer cells rely on testosterone to help them grow. Hormone therapy (also known as androgen deprivation therapy [ADT] or androgen suppression therapy) stops the body from producing testosterone or stops testosterone from reaching prostate cancer cells, which often makes prostate cancers shrink or grow more slowly for a time.

Hormone therapy for prostate cancer – continued

Hormone therapy alone, however, does not cure prostate cancer. Hormone therapy includes:

- **Orchiectomy** (surgical castration) – Surgical removal of the testicles, which reduces testosterone levels in the body quickly and significantly. This option is permanent and irreversible.
- **Drug therapy** (sometimes called chemical or medical castration)
  - **Luteinizing hormone-releasing hormone (LHRH) agonists and antagonists** – Medications that stop the body from producing testosterone.
    - LHRH agonist examples: Lupron, Eligard, Zoladex, Trelstar, Vantas
    - LHRH antagonist examples: Firmagon, Zytiga
  - **Anti-androgens** – Medications that block testosterone from reaching prostate cancer cells. They are usually given in conjunction with LHRH agonists, as LHRH agonists can cause a temporary increase in testosterone before levels decrease. Anti-androgen examples: Eulexin, Casodex, Nilandron, Xtandi
  - **Other medications** – When prostate cancer persists or recurs despite hormone therapy, other medications can be used to block testosterone in the body. Each medication targets testosterone in the body in a different way. Examples include corticosteroids such as prednisone and the anti-fungal drug ketoconazole.

Radioactive seed implantation

Radiation therapy for prostate cancer using implanted radioactive seeds is called brachytherapy. There are two types of brachytherapy:

- Permanent: Implanted seeds are left in place, but they become inert (no longer release radiation) after a period of weeks or months.
- Temporary: Seeds are implanted and left in place for about 30 minutes; the seeds and radioactive material then are removed.

The general consensus among respected sources is that, with permanent brachytherapy, the radioactive seeds are completely inactive in a year or less, and the cure rates are as effective as radical prostatectomy and external radiation.

Documentation tips for physicians

Overview

Documentation and coding of prostate cancer presents a special challenge, since most cases of prostate cancer are slow-growing and can be observed and monitored for many years with no active treatment. This situation may lead to vague documentation that in turn may lead to erroneous ICD-10-CM coding.

Current versus historical prostate cancer

- Do not use the phrase "history of" to describe current prostate cancer. In diagnosis coding, "history of" means the condition is historical and no longer exists as a current problem.
- On the other hand, do not document a final diagnosis of simply "prostate cancer" to describe a historical prostate cancer that was previously excised or eradicated and for which there is:
  a) No active treatment, and
  b) No evidence of disease or recurrence.
  In this scenario, it is appropriate to document "history of prostate cancer" with details of past diagnosis and treatment.

Purpose of PSA blood testing

After successful treatment of prostate cancer that results in complete eradication of the disease, regular monitoring for recurrence typically continues and includes ongoing laboratory testing of PSA. Documentation of ongoing PSA monitoring by itself without evidence that the prostate cancer is still present does not clearly support current prostate cancer. A final impression and plan of "prostate cancer – check PSA" is vague and ambiguous; it does not clearly indicate current versus historical prostate cancer or the purpose of checking the PSA level.

Metastatic prostate cancer

The final diagnosis should clearly indicate the primary and secondary sites. Consider these examples:

Example 1	
Final diagnosis	Metastatic prostate cancer
Comment	This diagnostic statement is ambiguous. It is not completely clear whether the prostate is the primary or secondary site.

Example 2	
Final diagnosis	Primary prostate cancer metastatic to pelvic bone
Comment	This diagnostic statement clearly identifies the prostate as the primary site and the pelvic bone as the secondary site.

ICD-10-CM tips and resources for coders

Coding prostate cancer

Cancer or carcinoma of the prostate codes as follows:

- C61 Malignant neoplasm of prostate
- C79.82 Secondary malignant neoplasm, genital organs
- DØ7.5 Carcinoma in situ of prostate

Carefully review and follow all instructional notes.

Coding prostate cancer as current

- Generally, prostate cancer is coded as current when the medical record clearly documents active treatment directed to the cancer for the purpose of cure or palliation and/or when the record clearly shows prostate cancer is still present but:
  o Is unresponsive to treatment;
  o The current treatment plan is observation only or "watchful waiting"; or
  o The patient has refused any further treatment.

Coding prostate cancer as historical

Prostate cancer is coded as historical (Z85.46) after the prostate cancer has been excised or eradicated, there is no active treatment directed to the prostate cancer and there is currently no evidence of disease or recurrence. Encounter for follow-up examination after treatment for malignant neoplasm has been completed is coded as ZØ8. Carefully review and follow all instructional notes.

Metastatic prostate cancer

For a current diagnosis of "metastatic prostate cancer" without further specification – and no more definitive information regarding the primary versus secondary site is obtained upon review of the entire medical record – the prostate is coded as the primary site (C61) with the secondary/metastatic site unknown (C79.9).

References: American Cancer Society; American Hospital Association (AHA) Coding Clinic; ICD-10-CM Official Guidelines for Coding and Reporting; Mayo Clinic; MD Anderson Cancer Center; MedlinePlus; National Cancer Institute; WebMD

Clinical overview

Definition and background

RA is a chronic, systemic inflammatory disorder that primarily affects the joints, causing pain, swelling and stiffness. It is an autoimmune disease in which the body's immune system attacks the body's own tissues. While the inflammatory response of rheumatoid arthritis affects primarily joints, it is a systemic inflammatory disorder that can also impact organs, such as the skin, eyes, heart, lungs and blood vessels. Rheumatoid arthritis usually begins after age 40, but it can occur at any age.

Causes

The exact cause of rheumatoid arthritis is not known. Some of the possible causes include:

- Genetic factors (inherited from parent to child)
- Environmental triggers
- Hormones (this disease is more common in women)

Signs and symptoms

Some people with this disease experience periods in which symptoms get worse (flares) or better (remissions). Others have a severe form of the disease that is active most of the time, lasts for many years or a lifetime and leads to serious joint damage and disability. Symptoms can include:

- Joint pain, warmth, redness and swelling
- Joint stiffness in the morning or after inactivity that can last for hours
- Fatigue
- Occasional fever
- Firm lumps (called rheumatoid nodules) that grow under the skin close to affected joints
- Loss of appetite and weight loss

Diagnostic tools

- Medical history and physical exam
- Evaluation by a rheumatologist (physician expert specially trained to diagnose, evaluate and treat rheumatic diseases)
- Joint X-rays
- Blood testing for inflammatory processes in the body or certain antibodies, for example:
    - Elevated erythrocyte sedimentation rate (also known as "ESR" or "sed rate") – indicates an inflammatory process
    - Rheumatoid factor or anti-cyclic citrullinated peptide (anti-CCP) – antibodies often found in patients with rheumatoid arthritis

Treatment

There is no cure for rheumatoid arthritis. The goal of treatment is to prevent joint damage, deformity and disability. With early and aggressive treatment, many patients can achieve long periods of time when inflammation is greatly reduced or absent with no active signs of disease (remission). The appropriate use of therapies is based on general principles that have been widely accepted by major working groups and by professional organizations of rheumatologists. These principles include:

1. Early recognition and diagnosis
2. Care by an expert in the treatment of rheumatic diseases, such as a rheumatologist
3. Early use of disease-modifying antirheumatic drugs (DMARDs) for all patients diagnosed with rheumatoid arthritis
4. Importance of tight control with target of remission or low disease activity
5. Use of anti-inflammatory agents, including nonsteroidal anti-inflammatory drugs (NSAIDs) and glucocorticoids, only as adjuncts to therapy

- **Drug therapy:** Many different types of drugs are used, often in combination. Examples:
    - **DMARDs** – relieve symptoms, slow disease progression and protect joints and other tissues from permanent damage. Examples: methotrexate, Plaquenil (hydroxychloroquine), Azulfidine (sulfasalazine), Arava (leflunomide), Minocin (minocycline)
    - **Immunosuppressants** – calm the immune system, which is attacking the body's own tissues. Examples: Imuran (azathioprine), Sandimmune (cyclosporine), Gengraf (cyclosporine)
    - **TNF-alpha inhibitors** – inhibit the action of tumor necrosis factor-alpha, which is an inflammatory substance produced by the body. Inhibiting this substance reduces the symptoms of rheumatoid arthritis. Examples: Enbrel (etanercept), Remicade (infliximab), Humira (adalimumab)
    - **Other drugs that target a variety of inflammatory processes** – Examples: Rituxan (rituximab), Orencia (abatacept), Kineret (anakinra)
- **Physical and occupational therapy**
- **Joint surgery** – if medications and conservative measures fail to prevent or slow joint damage.

Clinical overview

Self-management strategies

- Regular exercise and physical activity when symptoms are controlled
- Rest when joints are inflamed, with gentle range of motion and stretching
- Application of heat or cold
- Skilled relaxation techniques
- Disease-specific patient education
- Complementary and alternative therapies, such as acupuncture, biofeedback, yoga and dietary supplements, such as plant or fish oils

---

Rheumatoid arthritis versus osteoarthritis – A comparison by WebMD

Rheumatoid arthritis and osteoarthritis are different types of arthritis. They share some characteristics, but each has different symptoms and requires different treatment; thus, an accurate diagnosis is important.

Osteoarthritis is the most common form of arthritis. Rheumatoid arthritis affects only about one-tenth as many people as osteoarthritis does. The main difference between osteoarthritis and rheumatoid arthritis is the cause behind the joint symptoms.

- Osteoarthritis is caused by mechanical wear and tear on joints.
- Rheumatoid arthritis is an autoimmune disease in which the immune system attacks the body's own joints.

	Rheumatoid arthritis	Osteoarthritis
Age of onset	May begin at any time in life	Usually begins later in life
Speed of onset	Relatively rapid, over weeks to months	Slow, over years
Joint symptoms	Pain, swelling, stiffness	Achiness and tenderness, but little or no swelling
Pattern of joints affected	Often affects small and large joints on both sides of the body (symmetrical), such as both hands, both wrists or elbows, or balls of both feet	Often begins on one side of the body and may spread to the other side. Symptoms begin gradually and are often limited to one set of joints, usually the finger joints closest to the fingernails or thumbs, large weight-bearing joints (hips, knees) or the spine.
Duration of morning stiffness	Longer than one hour	Less than one hour – returns at the end of the day or after periods of activity
Presence of symptoms affecting the whole body (systemic)	Frequent fatigue and a general feeling of being ill	Whole body symptoms are not present

---

Documentation tips for physicians

Abbreviations

A good rule of thumb for any medical record is to limit – or avoid altogether – the use of acronyms and abbreviations. While "RA" is a commonly accepted medical abbreviation for rheumatoid arthritis, this abbreviation can have other meanings. The meaning of an abbreviation can sometimes be determined based on context, but this is not always true.

Best practice:

- The first mention in the office note of any medical diagnosis should be spelled out in full with the abbreviation in parentheses, i.e., "rheumatoid arthritis (RA)."
- Subsequent mention can be made using the abbreviation, except in the final assessment, where the diagnosis should again be documented in full.

Establishing the diagnosis

- When a patient reports a history of rheumatoid arthritis, the physician or other health care provider must validate this diagnosis through review of prior medical records, diagnostic test results and consulting specialist reports.
- Document details of diagnostic work-up and the outcome of current rheumatology specialist consultations. Include the name of the consulting rheumatologist.

Subjective

- In the subjective section of the office note, document any current symptom of rheumatoid arthritis reported by the patient (joint pain, swelling or stiffness; fatigue; episodes of fever; etc.).
- If there are no current symptoms, this section should show the patient was screened for symptoms.

Objective

In the objective section of the office note, document:

- Any current associated physical exam finding (such as joint deformity, etc.)
- Related laboratory or diagnostic imaging test results

Final assessment/impression

- Describe rheumatoid arthritis with the highest specificity (seropositive, seronegative, the particular joints affected, laterality, current status – active versus remission).

Final assessment/impression – continued

- Clearly link associated conditions or manifestations of rheumatoid arthritis by using linking terms such as "with," "due to," "secondary to" and "associated with."
- Do not document rheumatoid arthritis as a confirmed condition if it is only suspected and not truly confirmed. Rather, document signs and symptoms in the absence of a confirmed diagnosis.
- If rheumatoid arthritis is a confirmed diagnosis, do not describe it with terms that imply uncertainty (such as "apparently," "likely," "consistent with," "probable," etc.).
- Rheumatoid arthritis that is in remission but was taken into consideration by the physician or other health care provider when evaluating and treating the patient:
  - Should not be described as "history of." (In diagnosis coding, the phrase "history of" implies a past condition that no longer exists as a current problem.)
  - Should not be documented only in the past medical history; rather, it should be included in the final impression/assessment.
  - Should be described as "rheumatoid arthritis in remission."

Treatment plan

Document a specific and concise treatment plan for RA.

DMARDs

The American College of Rheumatology advises that patients with an established diagnosis of rheumatoid arthritis should be treated with a DMARD, even in the first six months after the diagnosis, unless a contraindication, inactive disease or patient refusal is documented. Best documentation practices regarding DMARD therapy require the physician to document:

a) Specific details of current DMARD therapy in the treatment plan section of the record (not simply the medication list) with clear linkage of the medication to rheumatoid arthritis; or
b) Specific information describing any contraindication to DMARD therapy; or
c) A notation that rheumatoid arthritis is inactive; or
d) A statement of patient refusal of DMARD therapy and the reason for refusal.

ICD-10-CM tips and resources for coders

Coding rheumatoid arthritis

For accurate and specific diagnosis code assignment, the coder must:

- Review the entire medical record and note the exact rheumatoid arthritis description documented in the medical record; then, in accordance with ICD-10-CM official coding conventions and guidelines:
  a) Search the alphabetic index for that specific description.
  b) Verify the code in the tabular list, carefully following all instructional notes.

Rheumatoid arthritis and its associated disorders classify to the following categories:

- **MØ5** Rheumatoid arthritis with rheumatoid factor *Excludes1* rheumatic fever (IØØ); juvenile rheumatoid arthritis (MØ8.-); and rheumatoid arthritis of spine (M45.-)
- **MØ6** Other rheumatoid arthritis

  ➢ Fourth, fifth and sixth characters are used with categories MØ5 and MØ6 to further specify the type of rheumatoid arthritis, as well as the particular site (joint affected) with laterality (left, right or unspecified).

- As noted in the documentation section, while RA is a commonly accepted medical abbreviation for rheumatoid arthritis, this abbreviation can have other meanings (e.g., refractory anemia, reactive arthritis, risk assessment). The meaning of an abbreviation can sometimes be determined based on context, but this is not always true. Use caution when coding RA – this abbreviation should not be coded as rheumatoid arthritis unless the individual medical record clearly shows RA is being used to represent rheumatoid arthritis.
- Severe joint pain is a characteristic of rheumatoid arthritis and is not coded separately from an already confirmed rheumatoid arthritis diagnosis.
- Do not code rheumatoid arthritis as a confirmed condition if it is documented as suspected and not truly confirmed. Rather, code the signs and symptoms in the absence of a confirmed diagnosis.

Rheumatoid arthritis in remission

RA documented as in remission is coded as current.

Seropositive versus seronegative rheumatoid arthritis

In most cases of rheumatoid arthritis, the patient's blood tests positive for rheumatoid factor and/or certain other antibodies (anti-CCP antibodies). These positive blood tests indicate the patient has seropositive rheumatoid arthritis, meaning the patient possesses the antibodies that cause an attack on joints and lead to inflammation.

- Seropositive rheumatoid arthritis codes to category MØ5 with fourth, fifth and sixth characters to provide further specificity, including site and laterality.

Patients can develop rheumatoid arthritis without the presence of these antibodies. This is referred to as seronegative rheumatoid arthritis. Seronegative patients are those who do not test positive for rheumatoid factor or anti-CCPs.

- Seronegative rheumatoid arthritis codes to category MØ6 with fourth, fifth and sixth characters to provide further specificity, including site and laterality.

Long-term (current) use of immunosuppressant drugs

- ICD-10-CM does not provide a specific code to identify long-term use of immunosuppressant drugs. Assign code Z79.899, other long-term (current) drug therapy, to report long-term use of immunosuppressant drugs.
- Do not assign a code for an immunocompromised state caused by drug treatment of rheumatoid arthritis. Immunosuppressant drugs are commonly used in the treatment of autoimmune diseases such as rheumatoid arthritis for the specific purpose of suppressing the immune system.

References: American College of Rheumatology; American Hospital Association Coding Clinic; Arthritis Foundation; ICD-10-CM Official Guidelines for Coding and Reporting; Mayo Clinic; National Center for Complementary and Alternative Medicine; National Institute of Arthritis and Musculoskeletal and Skin Diseases

Clinical overview

Definitions

- **Seizure**: An abnormal electrical discharge in the brain caused by clearly identifiable external factors that may be resolved or reversed (e.g., injury, high fever, substance abuse, metabolic disorders). An isolated seizure or an isolated episode of seizures without recurrence is not considered to be epilepsy.
- **Epilepsy, also known as seizure disorder**: A chronic brain disorder characterized by recurrent (two or more) seizures on more than one occasion that are not provoked by a clearly identifiable external factor. Epileptic seizures range from clinically undetectable to convulsions. The symptoms vary depending on the part of the brain involved in the epileptic discharge.
  - **Intractable epilepsy**: Epilepsy that does not respond to treatment.
  - **Status epilepticus**: A potentially life-threatening state in which a person experiences an abnormally prolonged seizure (any seizure lasting longer than five minutes) or does not fully regain consciousness between seizures. This condition represents a medical emergency.
- **Convulsion:** A sudden, uncontrollable and rapid shaking of the body caused by repeated contraction and relaxation of voluntary muscles.

Even though the terms "seizures" and "epilepsy" are sometimes used interchangeably, they are not one and the same. A seizure occurs when there is disorganized and chaotic electrical activity within the brain. This means a seizure is a sign or symptom of miscommunication between brain cells due to this abnormal electrical activity in the brain. By contrast, epilepsy (also called seizure disorder) is a precise medical condition that produces seizures affecting a variety of mental and physical functions. When a person has two or more unprovoked seizures, he or she is considered to have epilepsy.

Causes

The cause may be unknown (idiopathic). Known causes include, but are not limited to:

- Hereditary factors
- Traumatic brain injury
- Stroke or transient ischemic attack
- Congenital brain defects or birth injuries
- Drug overdose
- High fever
- Alcohol or drug abuse or withdrawal
- Brain infections, such as meningitis or encephalitis

Types of seizures/signs and symptoms

Seizures are divided into two major categories:

1) **Partial seizures** (also known as focal seizures) occur in just one part of the brain. They are frequently described by the area of the brain where they originate (e.g., focal frontal lobe seizure). Types:
   - **Simple partial seizure** – The person remains conscious but has altered emotions or sensations, such as sudden and unexplainable feelings of joy, anger, sadness, etc., or the person may hear, smell, taste, see or feel things that are not real.
   - **Complex partial seizure** – The person experiences altered or loss of consciousness, displaying strange, repetitious behaviors, such as blinks, twitches, mouth movements, etc. The person may experience auras (sensations that warn of an impending seizure).
2) **Generalized seizures** involve all of the brain. There are four types:
   - **Absence seizures (previously petit mal)** – brief loss of consciousness, staring, subtle body movements
   - **Myoclonic seizures** – jerks or twitches of the extremities
   - **Atonic seizures** – loss of muscle tone with sudden collapse or falling down
   - **Tonic-clonic seizures (previously grand mal)** – most intense symptoms, including loss of consciousness, stiffening and jerking of the body, loss of bladder control

Diagnostic tools

- Medical history and physical exam
- Electroencephalogram (EEG) (tests for abnormal electrical activity in the brain)
- Blood tests to check for metabolic imbalances
- Neuropsychological testing
- CT scan, PET scan and MRI to check for abnormalities in brain structure

Treatment

- Treatment or elimination of underlying cause, if known
- Medications (anticonvulsants)
- Identification and avoidance of triggers
- Dietary changes
- Various types of surgical intervention
- Implantation of vagus nerve or brain stimulator

Documentation tips for physicians

Abbreviations

A good rule of thumb for any medical record is to limit – or avoid altogether – the use of abbreviations. Commonly used abbreviations include SZ – seizure; AS – absence seizure; TLE – temporal lobe epilepsy; MTLE – medial temporal lobe epilepsy; and GTC – generalized tonic-clonic seizures. The meaning of an abbreviation can sometimes be determined based on context; however, this is not always true.

- Best practice is to always clearly spell out and fully describe the particular type of seizure, seizure disorder or epilepsy that is present.

Subjective

- In the subjective section of the office note, document the presence or absence of any current symptom related to seizure, seizure disorder, epilepsy, etc.

Objective

In the objective section of the office note, document:
- Any current associated physical exam finding
- Any related diagnostic test result

Final assessment/impression

- As noted above, best practice is to always clearly spell out and fully describe the particular type of seizure, seizure disorder or epilepsy that is present.
- Do not describe current seizure, seizure disorder or epilepsy as "history of." In diagnosis coding, the phrase "history of" means the condition is historical and no longer exists as a current problem.
- Do not document past seizures as current if they have resolved, have not recurred and are no longer being treated.
- Do not use terms that imply uncertainty ("probable," "apparently," "likely," "consistent with," etc.) to describe a current, confirmed seizure, seizure disorder or epilepsy.
- Do not document suspected and unconfirmed seizures, seizure disorder or epilepsy as if the condition were confirmed. Document signs and symptoms in the absence of a confirmed diagnosis.
- Document the current status of seizures, seizure disorder or epilepsy (stable, improved, worsening, historical with no recurrence, etc.).

Treatment plan

Document a specific and concise treatment plan for seizure, seizure disorder or epilepsy.
- Clearly link medications to the seizure or epilepsy diagnosis.
- Document planned diagnostic testing.
- If referrals are made or consultations requested, the office note should indicate to whom or where the referral or consultation is made or from whom consultation advice is requested.
- Document when the patient will be seen again.

Documentation and coding examples

Example 1	
Medical record documentation	Past medical history includes "seizures"
Medication list	Includes Topamax
Final assessment	Hypertension, hyperlipidemia, migraine headaches
ICD-10-CM codes	I1Ø Essential (primary) hypertension E78.5 Hyperlipidemia, unspecified G43.9Ø9 Migraine, unspecified, not intractable, without status migrainosus
Comments	No code is assigned for seizures, as this diagnosis is documented as a historical condition and is not supported as current. Topamax is an antiseizure medication, but it is not linked to any particular diagnosis. Further, Topamax can be used to treat migraine headaches – a diagnosis documented in the final assessment.

Example 2	
Final diagnosis	Symptomatic partial complex epilepsy localized to the right temporal lobe
ICD-10-CM code	G4Ø.2Ø9 Localization-related (focal) (partial) symptomatic epilepsy and epileptic syndromes with complex partial seizures, not intractable, without status epilepticus

ICD-10-CM tips and resources for coders

Coding basics

There are many different types of seizures, convulsions and epilepsy. Accurate code assignment is dependent on review of the entire medical record and the specific description of the condition. This is followed by location of the appropriate code in the alphabetic index and verification of the code in the tabular list with application of all instructional notes as appropriate.

Multiple abbreviations may be used to refer to seizures, seizure disorder, epilepsy, etc. A diagnosis code should not be assigned unless the meaning of the abbreviation is clear.

A diagnosis of epilepsy can have serious legal and personal implications for the patient (for example, inability to obtain a driver's license); therefore, a code for epilepsy must not be assigned unless the record clearly identifies the condition as such.

When the physician mentions a history of seizure in the workup but does not include any mention of seizures in the diagnostic statement, no code should be assigned unless clear documentation indicates that the criteria for reporting the condition have been met and the physician agrees that a code should be added.

Category R56, convulsions not elsewhere classified

Seizures or convulsions that are not identified as epilepsy or as a seizure disorder classify to category R56.

Category R56 appears in the tabular list of the ICD-10-CM manual under Chapter 18 – Symptoms, Signs and Abnormal Clinical and Laboratory Findings.

- Chapter 18 includes symptoms, signs and abnormal results of clinical or other investigative procedures and ill-defined conditions for which no diagnosis classifiable elsewhere is recorded.
- Category R56 requires fourth and fifth characters to specify the particular types of seizures or convulsions.

Some of the terms that classify to the sign/symptom category R56 are:

- Febrile convulsion(s)
- Febrile seizure
- Convulsive disorder
- Post-traumatic convulsion(s)
- Fit(s)
- Recurrent convulsions
- Seizure(s)

Category G4Ø, epilepsy and recurrent seizures

Category G4Ø appears in the tabular list of ICD-10-CM under Chapter 6 – Diseases of the Nervous System.

- Conditions in category G4Ø represent specific and precise diagnoses rather than a sign or symptom of another ill-defined disease or condition.
- Fourth and fifth characters are added to specify the particular type of epilepsy or recurrent seizures and whether the condition is intractable and with or without status epilepticus.

Terms such as "pharmacoresistant (pharmacologically resistant)," "poorly controlled," "refractory (medically)" and "treatment resistant" are considered equivalent to intractable. The coder should not assume the condition is intractable from general statements in the record.

Some of the terms that classify to the epilepsy and recurrent seizures category G4Ø are:

- Seizure disorder
- Epileptic attack
- Epileptic convulsion(s)
- Epileptic seizure(s)
- Epileptic fit
- Epilepsy

Post-traumatic seizures/post-traumatic epilepsy

A post-traumatic seizure is an initial or recurrent seizure that occurs during the acute phase following a traumatic brain injury and has no other known cause.

- Post-traumatic seizures code to R56.1, which **Excludes1** post-traumatic epilepsy (G4Ø.-)

Post-traumatic epilepsy is characterized by late seizures that occur more than a week after initial trauma. Late seizures are considered to be unprovoked, while early seizures (those occurring within a week of trauma) are considered to be provoked (those with an immediately identifiable cause, i.e., a direct result of the injury).

- For post-traumatic epilepsy, assign the appropriate epilepsy code based on the documented description followed by the appropriate code to report the traumatic condition with sequela.

Anti-epilepsy and anti-seizure medications

Many medications are used to treat conditions other than epilepsy or seizures. A coder cannot make assumptions when reviewing the medication list.

References: American Academy of Neurology; American Hospital Association Coding Clinic; Centers for Disease Control and Prevention; Epilepsy Foundation; ICD-10-CM and ICD-10-PCS Coding Handbook; ICD-10-CM Official Guidelines for Coding and Reporting; Mayo Clinic; MedlinePlus; Merck Manual; National Institute of Neurological Disorders and Stroke

Clinical overview

Background

The sinus node (also known as the sinoatrial node or SA node) is an area of specialized cells located in the right upper chamber of the heart (the right atrium).

- The cells of the sinus node generate regular electric impulses at a steady rate that spread through the upper chambers of the heart (the atria) and the lower pumping chambers (the ventricles) and cause the muscular contractions responsible for the pumping function of the heart.
- The electrical signals of the sinus node control the heart rate at a steady rate; thus, the sinus node is called the "natural pacemaker of the heart."
- Under normal conditions, the sinus node produces 60 to 100 impulses a minute, which is the normal resting heart rate.
- The sinus node can increase the heart rate during periods of stress, such as exercise or high fever.
- During quiet times, such as during sleep, the sinus node may slow down to below 60 impulses, or beats, per minute.

Definition

Sick sinus syndrome (SSS) is an abnormality or malfunction of the sinus node. The result is that the heart rate is no longer controlled at a regular rate and rhythm, and abnormal heart rhythms (arrhythmias) occur.

Types

- Sinoatrial block: Electrical signals pass too slowly through the sinus node, resulting in an abnormally slow heart rate.
- Sinus arrest: Sinus node activity pauses.
- Bradycardia-tachycardia syndrome: Heart rate alternates between abnormally fast and slow, sometimes with long pauses in between.

Causes

- Age-related wear and tear to the heart muscle (the most common cause)
- Diseases that cause damage to the heart's electrical system
- Medications

Signs and symptoms

- Pulse that is slower than normal
- Dizziness or lightheadedness
- Fainting or near fainting
- Shortness of breath
- Fatigue
- Chest pain
- Palpitations
- Confusion or memory problems
- Difficulty sleeping

There may be no symptoms.

Diagnostic tools

- Medical history and physical exam
- Standard electrocardiogram (ECG or EKG)
- Holter monitoring
- Cardiac event recording
- Electrophysiologic studies (EP studies)

Treatment

When there are no symptoms:

- Monitoring and regular follow-up

For symptomatic sick sinus syndrome:

- Medication management
- Implantation of a pacemaker
- Surgical procedures, such as ablation procedures that destroy small areas of cardiac tissue and disrupt the electrical impulses that are causing the problem

Documentation tips for physicians

Abbreviations

A good rule of thumb for a medical record is to limit — or avoid altogether – the use of abbreviations. While "SSS" is a commonly accepted medical abbreviation for sick sinus syndrome, best documentation practice is as follows:

- The initial notation of an abbreviation or acronym should be spelled out in full with the abbreviation/acronym in parentheses — e.g., "sick sinus syndrome (SSS)."
- Subsequent mention of the condition can be made using the abbreviation or acronym.

Subjective

The subjective section of the office note should document the presence or absence of any current signs or symptoms related to sick sinus syndrome (e.g., fatigue, dizziness, shortness of breath, etc.).

Objective

The objective section should include any current associated physical exam findings (abnormally slow or fast heart rate, low blood pressure, etc.) and related diagnostic testing results (abnormal heart rhythm on electrocardiogram, Holter monitor results, pacemaker interrogation and reprogramming, etc.).

Final assessment/impression

- Document current sick sinus syndrome by spelling it out in full.
- Do not describe current sick sinus syndrome as "history of." In diagnosis coding, the phrase "history of" means the condition is historical and no longer exists as a current problem.
- Do not use terms that imply uncertainty ("probable," "apparently," "likely," "consistent with," etc.) to describe current, confirmed sick sinus syndrome.
- Do not document suspected and unconfirmed sick sinus syndrome as if the condition were confirmed. Instead, document signs and symptoms in the absence of a confirmed diagnosis.
- Document the current status of sick sinus syndrome (stable, worsening, etc.).

Treatment plan

Document a specific and concise treatment plan for sick sinus syndrome.

- Document planned diagnostic testing.
- If referrals are made or consultations requested, the office note should indicate to whom or where the referral or consultation is made or from whom consultation advice is requested.
- Document when patient will be seen again.

Pacemaker documentation

Historically, the diagnosis coding authority – the American Hospital Association (AHA) Coding Clinic – has advised that when sick sinus syndrome is being controlled by a pacemaker and no problems are detected during routine pacemaker interrogation, no code is assigned for sick sinus syndrome. Depending on the specific circumstances documented in the medical record, it may be appropriate to assign one of these codes:

- Z45.Ø1Ø Encounter for checking and testing of cardiac pacemaker pulse generator (battery)
- Z45.Ø18 Encounter for adjustment and management of other part of cardiac pacemaker

Thus, when a pacemaker is present, it is imperative that the medical record clearly document whether:

a) The pacemaker is controlling the bradyarrhythmias associated with sick sinus syndrome;

b) Any problem with the pacemaker was detected;

c) Any medication is being used in addition to the pacemaker to control tachyarrhythmias associated with sick sinus syndrome (with clear linkage between the medication and the diagnosis/condition for which the medication is being used).

ICD-10-CM tips and resources for coders

Coding basics

For accurate and specific code assignment, the coder must:

a) Review the entire medical record to verify sick sinus syndrome is a current condition and not historical.

b) Note the exact description of sick sinus syndrome or related condition documented in the medical record; then, in accordance with ICD-10-CM official coding conventions and guidelines:

c) Search the alphabetic index for that specific description.

d) Verify the code in the tabular list, carefully following all instructional notes.

Coding sick sinus syndrome

Sick sinus syndrome classifies to code I49.5, which includes tachycardia-bradycardia syndrome. Code I49.5 falls under category I49, Other cardiac arrhythmias.

The diagnosis "sinoatrial node dysfunction" also codes to I49.5.

Category I49 **Excludes1** the following:
- Bradycardia NOS (RØØ.1)
- Neonatal dysrhythmia (P29.1-)
- Sinoatrial bradycardia (RØØ.1)
- Sinus bradycardia (RØØ.1)
- Vagal bradycardia (RØØ.1)

An **Excludes1** note indicates the code excluded should not be used at the same time as the code above the **Excludes1** note.

A diagnosis described as "sinus bradycardia" is not the same condition as sick sinus syndrome. Sinus bradycardia with no further description or specification simply means a slow heart rate. For sinus bradycardia to be coded as sick sinus syndrome, it must be described with terms that classify the condition to code I49.5 (for example, tachycardia-bradycardia syndrome).

Sick sinus syndrome with pacemaker

Pacemaker interrogation is a routine computer evaluation of pacemaker function. Pacemaker interrogation is routinely performed to verify the device is programmed accurately and to assess battery and lead function. Pacemaker settings may be reprogrammed if indicated.

Sick sinus syndrome with pacemaker – continued

In the past, AHA Coding Clinic (Sick sinus syndrome with pacemaker interrogation, Third Quarter 2010, Pages 9-10) has advised that when sick sinus syndrome is being controlled by the pacemaker and no problems are detected during routine pacemaker interrogation, no code is assigned for sick sinus syndrome. Depending on the specific circumstances documented in the medical record, it may be appropriate to assign one of these codes:

- Z45.Ø1Ø Encounter for checking and testing of cardiac pacemaker pulse generator (battery)
- Z45.Ø18 Encounter for adjustment and management of other part of cardiac pacemaker

Sick sinus syndrome can be coded as a current condition only when documented as a continuing and ongoing problem. When a pacemaker is present, sick sinus syndrome is not coded unless the medical record documentation shows:

a) Any associated bradyarrhythmia (slow heart rate) is not controlled by the pacemaker; and/or

b) Medications are being used to control any tachyarrhythmia (fast heart rate) associated with sick sinus syndrome (with documented linkage between the medication and the sick sinus syndrome diagnosis for which the medication is being used).

References: American Hospital Association Coding Clinic; ICD-10-CM Official Guidelines for Coding and Reporting; Mayo Clinic; MedlinePlus

Clinical overview

Definition

The bones of the spinal column are called vertebrae (plural) (vertebra – singular). A vertebral fracture is a break in a bone of the spine.

Types

- **Compression fracture** – Vertebral bone tissue collapses within itself, becoming squashed or compressed.
- **Burst fracture** – A more severe form of compression fracture in which the vertebra breaks in multiple directions.
- **Vertebral fracture-dislocation** – An unstable injury involving bone and/or soft tissue in which a vertebra moves off an adjacent vertebra (displacement). This type of injury can cause serious spinal cord compression.

Causes

Vertebral fractures can be traumatic, pathologic or both.

- **Traumatic** – caused by trauma or injury (for example, a patient falls and lands on his or her feet or buttocks. This causes downward pressure on the spinal column. The downward compressive force on the spine may be too great for the vertebrae to handle, causing one or more of the vertebrae to fracture.)
- **Pathologic** – caused by a disease process that weakens the bone, for example:
  - Osteoporosis (most common cause)
  - Tumors/cancers that started in the bones of the spine or tumors/cancers that started in other parts of the body and then spread to the bones of the spine
  - Other disease processes that weaken the bones of the spinal column
- **Both** – occurs when the bones of the spine are weakened by a disease process to the point that even minor injury or trauma causes a compression fracture. (Only the physician can determine that a fracture is out of proportion to the degree of trauma and is considered pathologic.)

Diagnostic tools

- Medical history and physical exam
- Imaging tests: spine X-ray, CT scanning and MRI
- Bone density testing for osteoporosis

Symptoms

There may be no symptoms. Symptoms may include:
- Back pain with sudden or chronic onset
- Loss of height
- Hunchback (kyphosis), which can occur with multiple fractures. (Kyphosis can cause pressure on the spinal cord that can rarely cause neurological symptoms, such as numbness, tingling or weakness; problems with walking; or problems with bowel or bladder function.)

Treatment

- Pain medications
- Bed rest
- Back bracing (sometimes used)
- Physical therapy
- Surgery
- Treatment of underlying condition (if pathologic fracture)

Potential complications

Complications can occur related to bed rest and immobility, such as:
- Blood clots
- Pulmonary embolism
- Pneumonia
- Pressure ulcers

Some of the surgical complications that can occur:
- Bleeding
- Infection
- Spinal fluid leaks
- Instrument failure
- Malunion
- Nonunion

Sequelae/late effects

A sequela (sequelae – plural) is a late effect – a residual condition produced after the acute phase of an illness or injury has ended. The sequela/residual condition may be apparent early or it may occur months or years later. Examples of sequelae of vertebral fractures include kyphosis (hunchback), spinal stenosis, prolonged chronic pain and spinal arthritis.

Prognosis

Most traumatic fractures heal in eight to 10 weeks with conservative treatment. Healing time will be slower if surgery is performed. Fractures related to osteoporosis usually become less painful with conservative management, but sometimes chronic pain and disability occur. The prognosis for vertebral compression fractures due to tumors depends on the type of tumor involved.

Documentation tips for physicians

Subjective

In the subjective section of the office note, document any current symptom related to vertebral fracture(s).

Objective

The objective section of the office note should include current associated physical exam findings and results of neurological testing and diagnostic imaging.

Final assessment/impression

- Use all applicable descriptors, as in:

Specific vertebral location (site/level)	Wedge compression	Unstable burst
Acute	Chronic	Stable burst
Displaced	Nondisplaced	Collapsed
Traumatic	Nontraumatic	Pathologic
Open	Closed	

- Document the cause of the fracture(s).
  - If traumatic, specify the type of injury or trauma, and when the injury occurred, if known.
  - If pathologic, clearly link the fracture to the underlying causative disease process. ALERT: In the ICD-10-CM classification, there is no default to either traumatic or pathological. Coders are advised to query the physician for clarification when the documentation does not clearly indicate whether the fracture is traumatic or pathological.
- Do not use the descriptor "history of" to describe a current vertebral fracture. In diagnosis coding, the phrase "history of" means the condition is historical and no longer exists as a current problem.
- A past vertebral fracture that has healed and no longer exists should not be documented in the final impression as if it is still current. In this scenario, it is appropriate to use the descriptor "history of."
- Do not document a suspected vertebral fracture as if it were confirmed. Rather, document the signs and symptoms in the absence of a confirmed diagnosis.
- For a confirmed current vertebral fracture, do not use descriptors that imply uncertainty (such as "probable," "apparently," "likely" or "consistent with").
- Document the current status (improving, unchanged, healed, etc.; or with complications such as delayed healing, nonunion or malunion).

Episode of care

The encounter note should clearly indicate the episode of care (i.e., initial, subsequent or sequela). Include the date of initial evaluation and a chronology of diagnosis and treatment of the fracture. See seventh-character descriptions on the following pages.

Treatment plan

Document a specific and concise treatment plan.

- If referrals are made or consultations requested, the office note should indicate to whom or where the referral or consultation is made or from whom consultation advice is requested.
- Document when the patient will be seen again.

Documentation and coding examples

Example 1	
Final diagnosis	Age-related osteoporosis with newly diagnosed L1 and L2 lumbar wedge compression fractures
ICD-10-CM code	M8Ø.Ø8xA Age-related osteoporosis with current pathological fracture, vertebra(e), initial encounter for fracture

Example 2	
Final diagnosis	Severe lumbar spinal stenosis due to history of traumatic wedge compression fractures of fourth and fifth lumbar vertebrae
ICD-10-CM codes	M48.Ø61 Spinal stenosis, lumbar region S32.Ø4ØS Wedge compression fracture of fourth lumbar vertebra, sequela S32.Ø5ØS Wedge compression fracture of fifth lumbar vertebra, sequela

Example 3	
Final diagnosis	Routine follow-up visit for healing T2 pathological vertebral fracture
ICD-10-CM code	M84.48xD Pathological fracture, other site, subsequent encounter for fracture with routine healing

Example 4	
Final diagnosis	Severe thoracolumbar kyphosis due to past thoracic and lumbar vertebral compression fractures
ICD-10-CM codes	M4Ø.15 Other secondary kyphosis, thoracolumbar region M48.48xS Pathological fracture, other site, sequela of fracture.

ICD-10-CM tips and resources for coders

Coding basics

For accurate and specific diagnosis code assignment, the coder must:

- Review the entire medical record.
- Note the exact description of the vertebral fracture(s) documented in the medical record; then, according to ICD-10-CM official coding conventions and guidelines:
  a) Search the alphabetic index for that specific description.
  b) Verify the code in the tabular list, carefully following all instructional notes.

The principles of multiple coding of injuries should be followed in coding fractures.

A fracture not indicated as open or closed is coded to closed. A fracture not indicated whether displaced or not displaced is coded to displaced. Multiple fractures are sequenced in accordance with the severity of the fracture.

Traumatic vertebral fractures

Traumatic vertebral fractures are coded in accordance with the provisions within categories S12, S22 and S32 and the level of detail documented in the medical record.

Traumatic vertebral fractures classify as follows:

Vertebral level	Subcategories
Cervical	S12.ØØ – S12.69
Thoracic	S22.ØØ – S22.Ø8
Lumbar	S32.Ø – S32.Ø5
Sacral	S32.1Ø – S32.19
Coccyx	S32.2

These subcategories include multiple instructional notes that must be carefully reviewed and applied as appropriate.

Fifth and sixth characters specify the particular site within each vertebral region of the spinal column and the type of fracture. There are many descriptors within each subcategory. A seventh character is added to specify the encounter as follows:

A: initial encounter for closed fracture
B: initial encounter for open fracture
D: subsequent encounter for fracture with routine healing
G: subsequent encounter for fracture with delayed healing
K: subsequent encounter for fracture with nonunion
S: sequela

Initial encounter – active treatment of traumatic vertebral fracture (seventh characters A and B)

- Seventh characters A and B are used for each encounter in which the patient is receiving active treatment for traumatic vertebral fracture (including patients who delayed seeking treatment for the fracture or nonunion):
  A: Initial encounter for closed fracture
  B: Initial encounter for open fracture
- Examples of active treatment: surgical treatment, emergency department encounter, evaluation and continuing (ongoing) active treatment by the same or a different physician.

While a patient may be seen by a new or different physician over the course of treatment for an injury, assignment of the seventh character is based on whether the patient is undergoing active treatment and not whether the physician is seeing the patient for the first time.

Subsequent encounter – routine aftercare of traumatic vertebral fracture (seventh character D)

This describes care given after the patient has completed active treatment of the fracture and is receiving routine care for the fracture during the healing or recovery phase. The seventh-character extension is:

D: subsequent encounter for fracture with routine healing

Examples of routine traumatic fracture aftercare: brace adjustment, X-ray to check healing status of fracture, medication adjustment and follow-up visits that occur after active fracture treatment has been completed.

The aftercare Z codes should not be used for aftercare for traumatic fractures.

Complications of traumatic vertebral fracture – seventh characters G and K

Care for complications of surgical treatment of traumatic vertebral fracture repairs during the healing or recovery phase are reported with the appropriate complication codes. Care of complications such as delayed union and nonunion is reported with seventh characters as follows:

G: subsequent encounter for fracture with delayed healing
K: subsequent encounter for fracture with nonunion

ICD-10-CM tips and resources for coders

Complications of traumatic vertebral fracture – seventh characters G and K (continued)

For complication codes, active treatment refers to treatment for traumatic vertebral fracture described by the code, even though it may be related to an earlier vertebral fracture. For example:

Code T84.63xA, infection and inflammatory reaction due to internal fixation device of spine, initial encounter, is used when active treatment is provided for the infection, even though the condition relates to the internal fixation device of the spine that was placed at a previous encounter.

Sequela of traumatic vertebral fracture – seventh character S

A sequela is a late effect – a residual condition produced after the acute phase of a vertebral fracture has ended. There is no time limit on when a sequela code can be used. The sequela may be apparent early, or it may occur months or years later. Sequelae are reported with seventh-character assignment as follows:

S: sequela

- Examples include kyphosis, spinal stenosis, prolonged chronic pain and spinal arthritis.
- Use both the traumatic vertebral fracture code and the code for the sequela itself. S is added only to the fracture code, not the sequela code.
- The specific type of sequela (e.g., kyphosis) is sequenced first, followed by the fracture code.

Pathological vertebral fractures

Pathological vertebral fractures are coded according to the provisions within the following subcategories and the level of detail documented in the medical record.

M80.08	Age-related osteoporosis with current pathological fracture, vertebra(e) x7th
M80.88	Other osteoporosis with current pathological fracture, vertebra(e) x7th
M84.48	Pathological fracture, other site x7th
M84.58	Pathological fracture in neoplastic disease, other site x7th (code also underlying neoplasm)
M84.68	Pathological fracture in other disease, other site x7th (code also underlying condition)

Review and follow instructional notes as appropriate.

Pathological vertebral fractures – continued

As noted, each subcategory requires a sixth-character placeholder (x), plus a seventh character to specify the encounter as follows:

A: initial encounter for fracture

D: subsequent encounter for fracture with routine healing

G: subsequent encounter for fracture with delayed healing

K: subsequent encounter for fracture with nonunion

P: subsequent encounter for fracture with malunion

S: sequela

Pathological fracture due to neoplasm

- For pathological fracture due to a neoplasm, when the focus of treatment is the fracture, a code from subcategory M84.5, pathological fracture in neoplastic disease, should be sequenced first, followed by the code for the neoplasm.
- When the focus of treatment is the neoplasm with an associated pathological fracture, the neoplasm code should be sequenced first, followed by a code from M84.5 for the pathological fracture.

Initial encounter – active treatment of pathological vertebral fracture (seventh character A)

- As long as the patient is receiving active treatment for the fracture, apply the following seventh character:
  A: initial encounter for fracture

- Examples of active treatment: surgical treatment, emergency department encounter, evaluation and continuing treatment by the same or a different physician.

  While a patient may be seen by a new or different physician over the course of treatment, seventh-character assignment is based on whether the patient is undergoing active treatment and not whether the physician is seeing the patient for the first time.

Subsequent encounter – routine aftercare of pathological vertebral fracture (seventh character D)

This describes care given after the patient has completed active treatment of the fracture and is receiving routine care for the fracture during the healing or recovery phase. The seventh-character extension is:

D: subsequent encounter for fracture with routine healing

ICD-10-CM tips and resources for coders

Subsequent encounter – routine aftercare of pathological vertebral fracture (seventh character D) – continued

- Examples of routine pathological fracture aftercare: brace adjustment, X-ray to check healing status of fracture, medication adjustment, follow-up visits that occur after active fracture treatment has been completed.

Complications of pathological vertebral fracture – seventh characters G, K and P

- Care for complications of surgical treatment of pathological vertebral fracture during the healing or recovery phase should be coded with the appropriate complication codes.

- Care of complications of pathologic fractures are reported with the appropriate seventh character as follows:
  G: subsequent care with delayed union
  K: subsequent care with nonunion
  P: subsequent care with malunion

Sequela of pathological vertebral fracture (seventh character S)

A sequela is a late effect – a residual condition produced after the acute phase of a vertebral fracture has ended. There is no time limit on when a sequela code can be used. The sequela may be apparent early or it may occur months or years later. Sequelae are reported with seventh-character assignment as follows:
S: sequela

- Examples include kyphosis, spinal stenosis, prolonged chronic pain and spinal arthritis.
- Use both the pathological vertebral fracture code and the code for the sequela itself. S is added only to the fracture code, not the sequela code.
- The specific type of sequela (e.g., kyphosis) is sequenced first, followed by the fracture code.

History of vertebral fractures

A vertebral compression fracture that occurred in the past and for which there are no current symptoms, treatment, complications or sequelae is coded as follows:

Z87.31Ø	Personal history of (healed) osteoporosis fracture
Z87.311	Personal history of (healed) other pathologic fracture
Z87.81	Personal history of (healed) traumatic fracture

References: American Academy of Orthopaedic Surgeons; American Hospital Association Coding Clinic; ICD-10-CM Official Guidelines for Coding and Reporting; MedlinePlus

Made in United States
Orlando, FL
09 March 2023

30876043R00059